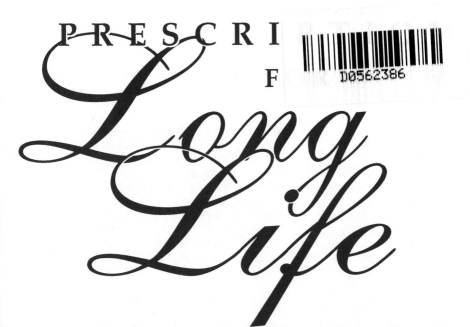

PRESCRI F Long Life

ESSENTIAL REMEDIES FOR LONGEVITY

DR. MITCHELL KURK
DR. MORTON WALKER

A DR. MORTON WALKER HEALTH BOOK

Avery Publishing Group
Garden City Park, New York

The medical information and procedures in this book are based upon the research, and personal and professional experiences, of the authors. The authors and publisher do not advocate the use of any particular form of health care but believe that the information presented in this book should be available to the public. This book is not intended to replace the advice and treatment of a physician.

Because there is always some risk involved, the authors and publisher are not responsible for any adverse effects or consequences resulting from the use of any of the preparations or procedures suggested in this book. Please do not use this book if you are unwilling to assume the risk. Each person and situation are unique, and a physician or other qualified health professional should be consulted if there is any question regarding the presence or treatment of any abnormal health condition. It is a sign of wisdom, not cowardice, to seek a second or third opinion.

The quotation on page 148 is from *Hydrogen Peroxide: Medical Miracle* by William Campbell Douglass. Reprinted by permission of Second Opinion Publishing.

Cover design: William Gonzalez
Typesetter: Al Berotti
In-house editor: Lisa James

Avery Publishing Group, Inc.
120 Old Broadway
Garden City Park, New York 11040
1-800-548-5757

Library of Congress Cataloging-in-Publication Data

Kurk, Mitchell.
    Prescription for long life : essential remedies for longevity /
Mitchell Kurk, Morton Walker.
        p.   cm.
    Includes bibliographical references and index.
    ISBN 0-89529-790-6 (pbk.)
        1. Longevity—Popular works.   2. Longevity—Physiological aspects.
I. Walker, Morton.   II. Title.
RA776.75.K87   1998
613—dc21   97-35936
                                                                      CIP

Printed in the United States of America

10   9   8   7   6   5   4   3

Contents

From Dr. Mitchell Kurk
To my wife, Marcia,
whose fatal illness led me into alternative medicine

From Dr. Morton Walker
To The Cancer Control Society's Executive Director,
Lorraine Rosenthal, whose dedication to alternative medicine
has benefited millions of people worldwide

Acknowledgments

From Dr. Mitchell Kurk: I wish to acknowledge my dear mother, who encouraged me to become a doctor; my office staff, especially Theresa John, for their long, dedicated, and tireless efforts to maintain my high standards of medical practice; and my editor, Lisa James, of Avery Publishing Group for her assistance in the final preparation of this manuscript.

Foreword

Early in 1980, a physician whom I had never met before walked into my office and asked to tour my treatment center in Huntington, New York. Mitchell Kurk, M.D., had recently returned from a place considered to be a source of the fountain of youth, the National Institute of Gerontologic Research and Geriatric Medicine in Bucharest, Rumania, directed by Anna Aslan, M.D. Dr. Aslan was renowned throughout Europe as a gerontologist, a doctor who specializes in the effects of aging.

Dr. Kurk and I spoke about his wonderful experiences with Dr. Aslan. We also discussed the things he learned in Bucharest, information that is included in this book, *Prescription for Long Life*. She had taught him how to produce his own formula for her injectible antiaging vitamin Gerovital, which had been banned from import into the United States by the U.S. Food and Drug Administration.

When explorer Juan Ponce de León went looking for his own fountain of youth in what is now Florida, he possibly knew about *Los Viejos* (the old ones) of Ecuador. The old ones drank of mineral-laden water, a fountain that Ponce de León had been seeking. As revealed in this book, coauthors Dr. Kurk and Morton Walker, D.P.M., a medical journalist specializing in wholistic medicine, discuss how a lack of essen-

tial minerals plays a major role in aging. The fountain of
youth is a cascade of many converging rivers represented by
different aspects of alternative medicine.

With much fanfare, for instance, mainstream medicine has
finally accepted that free radical pathology is at the core of
degenerative diseases and the accelerated aging process. Finally, conventional medical doctors have realized that cancer,
arthritis, cardiovascular disorders, and other conditions come
from diverse bombardments of free radicals. Of course, researchers such as Dr. Kurk and Dr. Walker have been stat-
ing this precept for more than thirty years. Stress, petro-
chemical residues, toxic fumes, malnourishing fast foods, and
poor lifestyles all accelerate the aging aspects of free radical
pathology.

In reading *Prescription for Long Life*, I realized that all of us
in wholistic medicine have come a long way. Dr. Kurk and
Dr. Walker are sharing their vast knowledge with you, and
this is an admirable attribute. The word "doctor" comes from
the Latin *docere*, which means "to teach." These two authors
deserve to be designated "doctor." They cover all aspects of
antiaging knowledge.

What appeals to me even more about this book is its general overview of alternative methods of healing. The term "alternative" has become a staple of today's medical language,
especially since it is associated with the Office of Alternative
Medicine at the National Institutes of Health. We who are alternative physicians dispense the oldest form of medical care,
in which the Hippocratic first law of medicine is *prima non
nocere*, or "first, do no harm."

In all honesty, conventional allopathic medicine cannot af-
firm that *prima non nocere* is the principle it always follows.
All of us have witnessed with dismay the side effects of aggressive intervention medicine. In contrast, the information offered in *Prescription for Long Life* gives you safer, better, more
natural techniques for keeping yourself in good health, over-
coming most disorders, and reversing disease processes.

Dr. Morton Walker and Dr. Mitchell Kurk present alterna-
tives such as chelation therapy, relaxation training, and an-

tioxidant therapies. They all play major roles in the reversal of ill health at relatively low cost. Also, these procedures don't involve high-tech equipment or body invasion.

Inasmuch as the modern fountain of youth is made up of many converging rivers, the authors present both home remedies and those that must be administered under medical supervision. At a time when medicine delivery and cost-effectiveness have come under scrutiny, all of us are collectively responsible for changing the current state of events through self-education.

So here you hold *Prescription for Long Life*, with its advice for improving your longevity. One can hope that you will act on what is taught in these pages. We know that you have a wish to learn. More than anyone else, you have the power to effect changes for the better in your body, mind, and emotions.

More than two thirds of all Americans have expressed the desire to employ alternative methods of healing, orthomolecular nutrition, and wholistic medicine, as shown in a significant survey conducted by the American Medical Association. In this book, the authors furnish this knowledge. They have provided you with a highly instructional tool that is easy to read and well illustrated with patient stories and examples. I wholeheartedly recommend *Prescription for Long Life*, not only for its antiaging aspects, but also as a general book about alternative medicine.

Serafina Corsello
Wholistic physician and medical director of
The Corsello Centers for Nutritional/Complementary Medicine

Preface

What makes me so certain that the human life span is far in excess of the actual one is this: Among all my autopsies (and I have performed quite a few), I have never seen a man who died of old age. In fact, I do not think anyone has ever died of old age yet. We invariably die because one vital part has worn out too early in proportion to the rest of the body.

—Hans Selye, M.D., Ph.D., D.Sc.
in *Stress Without Distress*, 1974

From the beginning of time, people have been trying to stave off aging, illness, and death. Now, with new insights into the aging process, humankind is much closer to achieving this goal. There are techniques and therapies that can help delay the biological signs of advancing age. With help from wholistic physicians, people are rediscovering the strength, vitality, and sexuality that they had known in youth.

Nobody knows for sure why we age, become sick, and die. Even without illness, nothing can stop the inherent genetic program that sets the course of our lives. Often, as people age, fat deposits accumulate, sexual appetites wane, brain cells die, arteries harden or become blocked, muscles lose resilience, and mechanisms for fighting off disease lose their potency.

While everyone ages, there are great differences in the speed at which the process occurs. Some people lose their full mental capacity early, while others retain their alertness and creativity into old age. Some people are afflicted with heart disease and arthritis, while others never are. Some people wrinkle early, while others retain a soft, smooth skin.

The reasons for these variations involve a combination of genetic and nongenetic factors. Some people have such hardy constitutions that they live to very old ages despite unfavorable living conditions. However, most people die before the end of their natural life spans because of environmental factors, such as pollution, and unhealthy habits that accelerate aging.

Medical science currently can do little to alter one's genetic program. However, physicians who practice wholistic medicine, such as Dr. Kurk, are exploring therapies that can slow down other aspects of the aging process. These therapies are offshoots of traditional medical methods, but are approached from a different point of view.

Many wholistic physicians start practicing alternative medicine after finding that conventional treatments did not always help their patients. For example, Dr. Kurk had spent years giving cortisone injections to his arthritic patients, only to find that the relief cortisone provided was temporary. He started administering procaine, a local anesthetic used most often in dentistry, after reading about a procaine-based anti-aging formula called Gerovital. His discovery that procaine improved his patients' overall health led him to study with Gerovital's inventor, Rumanian gerontologist Dr. Ana Aslan (see Chapter 17).

As time went on, Dr. Kurk became interested in helping his older patients regain the vitality they knew in youth. He encouraged them to lose weight if they needed to; become physically active; drop sugar from their diets; reduce their intake of salt, fat, and meat; take nutritional supplements; and follow other healthy practices. This led him to develop a complete program for youth extension. His program employs therapies that can help treat diseases such as arthritis, bronchial asthma, rheumatism, senile parkinsonism, and angina pectoris.

All of Dr. Kurk's research is in *Prescription for Long Life*. It comes from long experience with thousands of patients who have gained immeasurable benefits from this program. We trust that you will put this knowledge into practice so that you can discover these benefits for yourself.

Introduction

Have you ever asked yourself just how long your life will last and how healthy it will be? Many people say they want to live longer lives, but only if they can retain their health. This is an understandable concern. Almost everyone knows a person who suffered a drastic decline in physical and mental health toward the end of life. And even if the decline age brings is not drastic, it can still be frustrating. No one wants to see wrinkles develop or feel a loss of energy and vitality.

Age does not have to bring a decline in function. There are ways to slow the aging process. They can help you regain energy, revitalize your sex life, restore your memory, ease aches and pains, strengthen your body, and feel twenty years younger. Before we turn our attention to this topic, however, it would be a good idea to look at some statistics, and to see how an unconventional approach to medicine can help you live longer.

HOW LONG WILL YOUR LIFE LAST?

Average life spans have increased dramatically in the industrialized world over the course of the twentieth century. In 1900, people in North America survived to an average age of about 55. Today, the average life expectancy in the United States is 74.9 years—78.9 years for women and 72.0 years for men. More than 2.6 million Americans are now 85 years old or older. By the year 2040, this group will increase to more than 13 million. Medical science and improved public health measures have succeeded in eliminating or curing many diseases that once caused illness and early death, such as tuberculosis, smallpox, and poliomyelitis. (With the advent of AIDS, though, tuberculosis has again become a public health problem.)

While it is true that people in industrialized countries have enjoyed increasing longevity, they do seem to be aging faster. People in these countries develop degenerative diseases that disable their senior years, causing a deterioration in the quality of life. Many believe that it is almost better to die than to linger in discomfort and pain.

An increase in the rate at which people age is being borne out statistically. In thirty-four countries, life expectancy both at birth and at age sixty-five is greater in the developed nations, where medicine had overcome the plagues of childhood. This is to be expected. Of much greater significance is that a man's life expectancy today at age sixty-five is greater in Greece and Iceland than it is in the United States. Greece and Iceland are two of the Western world's least industrialized countries. In fact, twenty-three of the thirty-four nations reported a drop in the life expectancy of their 65-year-old population. With the single exception of Japan, this includes all of the world's highly industrialized nations.

This means that if you are fifty or sixty years old and live in North America, your life expectancy is less than it was for someone your age only ten or twenty years ago, according to the WHO statistics. This reduced longevity has occurred because of an increase in degenerative diseases such as high blood pressure, emphysema, cancer, cardiovascular ailments, and others. The elimination of heart disease alone would increase life expectancy at birth by more than twelve years for men and ten years for women. An American man's expected life span would thus be eighty-nine, if heart attack was no longer the single biggest cause of death.

Oddly enough, the prospects for living to a ripe old age—perhaps 120 years, the age for which human beings are genetically coded—are far better than they have ever been. You may not think a 120-year life span is possible. Yet, there are parts of the world where people do live such long lives. A census in Vilcabamba, one village in southern Ecuador, showed that out of little more than 800 inhabitants, about a dozen were more than 100 years old. These figures cannot be explained by genetics, since young Vilcabambans who left the village for the larger Ecuadorian cities suffered shortened life spans. (City dwellers in Ecuador die at about the same average age as Americans.)

Among the centenarians in Vilcabamba, blood serum cholesterol levels averaged as low as 140 mg/dl—about 80 points lower than that of the average "healthy" middle-aged American. Vilcabambans consume about 1,700 calories a day, of which only 153 calories are from animal fat. On average, an adult American man eats between 2,400 and 2,600 calories a day, of which 450 to 500 calories are from animal fat. As a result, diseases such as heart disease, diabetes, and cancer are almost unknown in Vilcabamba. Exercise, in the form of hard manual labor, also plays a big role in keeping Vilcabambans healthy, as does the relaxed pace of their daily existence. Of special importance is the presence of antiaging minerals in their drinking water.[1] (For more information on these remarkable people, see Chapter 17.)

WHOLISTIC MEDICINE AND WHAT IT MEANS FOR LONGEVITY

Conventional medicine has vastly improved the health of many people. It has found cures for infectious diseases. It has created body-imaging systems that allow doctors to diagnose problems earlier than ever before. It has developed sophisticated surgical techniques for transplanting vital organs and replacing worn-out joints.

Conventional medicine's greatest weakness, however, lies in disease prevention. It tends to see the patient as a collection of body systems, each of which is treated as a separate entity. Often, patients will see different doctors for different problems, and receive piecemeal, uncoordinated treatment as a result.

On the other hand, wholistic medicine treats the entire person, body and mind, as one unified entity. The practitioner of wholistic medicine may be likened to a potter. While the pot spins on the wheel, the potter is constantly examining it, using all of his or her aesthetic, artistic, and intuitive faculties as well as his logical faculties. He or she works with and molds the clay to keep it as perfectly symmetrical as possible. Should one area start to become asymmetrical, the potter rebalances and recenters the pot. The potter never works on only one area, but always on the entire pot.

That is the way it is with wholistic medical practice. The doctor tries to mold his or her patient's health by adjusting immune response to pollutants, carcinogens, allergens, and other sources of disease. The wholistic doctor also stresses the patient's responsibility for health, through such means as improved diet, proper exercise, and other measures.

If you are not functioning at a high level of wellness, you may benefit from wholistic medicine. To prolong your life, you must view yourself, not just as a biological machine, but as a unit made up of both body and mind. Both must be healthy for you to achieve your maximum life span.

Dr. Kurk practices wholistic medicine. This approach has led him to develop the antiaging techniques described in this book. In Part I, we discuss some causes of aging, including free radicals (Chapter 1), stress (Chapter 2), brain allergies (Chapter 3), and mineral toxicity or imbalance (Chapter 4). In Part II, we discuss Dr. Kurk's prescription for long life. This includes vitamin and mineral supplementation (Chapters 5 through 9), fiber (Chapter 10), internal cleansers (Chapter 11), yogurt (Chapter 12), chelation therapy (Chapter 13), herbal tonics (Chapter 14), intravenous hydrogen peroxide (Chapter 15), DHEA (Chapter 16), and an antiaging formula called Gerovital (Chapter 17). In Chapter 18, we use this information to create a total antiaging program.

This program has worked for Dr. Kurk's own patients. For example, sixty-one-year-old Robert A. of Pennsylvania used to be run down, fatigued all the time, filled with discomfort in his muscles and joints, and feeling that he had reached the end of the line. (As is the case with most of the other patients discussed in this book, "Robert A." is not his real name.) He would misplace his eyeglasses and car keys, and could not recall telephone numbers he frequently needed. He lived alone and often locked himself out of his apartment. Robert was worried.

Robert visited Dr. Kurk, who put the patient on a full stress-reduction program that included weight control, dietary improvement and supplementation, intravenous injections, daily exercises, and other procedures. A few weeks later, Robert came back—with his 28-year-old fiancée. Today, he and his wife have three children. He works forty-eight hours a week, runs marathons about three times a year, and enjoys vigorous daily exercise.

The benefits Robert has experienced—better health, enhanced sexuality, and greater stamina—are not unusual. Other people who have followed Dr. Kurk's advice have had the same results.

Both of us put this program to work in our own lives. Neither of us can say with certainty how long we'll live, but we do know we have a better chance of staying healthier longer. We think this program can help you live a longer, healthier life, too.

Part I

What Causes Aging

All of us think of growing old as a natural event, and indeed it is. And it is true that more Americans are living into their seventies, eighties, and nineties than ever before. But there is evidence that our natural life span can well exceed a century. Why doesn't it? In this part, we will look at four causes of premature aging—free radicals, stress, allergies, plus mineral toxicity and imbalances—and at how these conditions can damage our health and rob us of those extra years of life.

Chapter 1

The Free Radical Reason for Premature Aging

Are dry patches gradually appearing on your face and cheeks?
Are you developing growths on your skin, such as moles or skin tags?
Is your hair dry, brittle, or graying too soon?
Do your fingernails grow slowly and then break or peel?
Do your hands and feet frequently feel cold?
Do you bruise easily?
Do your gums bleed readily or bleed whenever you brush your teeth?

If you answer "yes" to more than one of these questions, it is likely that you are showing signs of premature aging. By giving you this series of minor signals, your body is trying to tell you something vitally important about how to prolong your life. If you don't become more aware of what you're doing wrong in terms of your lifestyle, your natural, built-in life span—as determined by the genetic code with which you were born—will be much shortened.

In this chapter, we'll first look at what scientists believe to be the maximum human life span. We'll then see how substances called free radicals can cause premature aging, and how these harmful substances can be neutralized by antioxidants.

THE PROBLEM OF AGING

Ever since humans began to think and dream sufficiently to inspire fantasies and myths, they have asked several intriguing questions: What causes us to grow old? What, if anything, can we do to slow this process? How must we proceed to have not only a longer life but a better quality of living, as well?

The only nonaging animal in the world is the sea anemone. It constantly replaces all its cells and is more nearly a culture of multiple organisms rather than a single organism. The rest of us age, but obtaining a precise, all-inclusive definition of aging is difficult. Some gerontologists, doctors who specialize in the problems associated with aging, define aging as progressive accumulation over time of changes responsible for increased susceptibility to disease and, finally, to death, the last event of advancing age. Others define aging as "a progressive deterioration of the organism after maturity of size or function has been reached and which is universal, intrinsic, progressive, and deleterious with time."[1]

In recent years, the questions surrounding age have inspired a significant body of scientific research on aging and longevity. Considering evidence that many important biological functions continue to work superbly for well over 100 years, the "normal" human life span is thought to be 120 to 150 years (see Chapter 17). Yet life expectancy in the United States now falls about 50 to 80 years short of those numbers. Forty percent of the factors affecting life expectancy can be controlled, according to gerontologists. They are suggesting that not only can length of life be extended but that quality of life can be maintained as well through better health maintenance.

The complex mechanism of the aging process and of the progressive accumulation of changes with time are unknown. However, many theories about the nature of the central cause of aging have been proposed.[2] One of these theories concerns free radical pathology. Aging research provides insights on how the body deteriorates because of free radical pathology, and on ways to possibly delay the aging process.[3]

FREE RADICAL THEORY OF AGING

A major theory of aging research, one that is becoming generally accepted as fact, suggests that *free radicals* damage body cells. This damage, in turn, causes the pathological changes associated with growing old.[4] Free radical production is related to the body's use of oxygen. Some of the oxygen in our bodies is converted into water. Usually, this conversion happens immediately. Sometimes, though, the process takes a little longer, and the oxygen can assume very unstable forms called peroxides until the process is completed. These unstable oxygen molecules tends to react with other molecules around them, which can result in severe damage to cells, specifically to the cells' membranes. Such damage may disrupt various processes within the body.

While free radicals are normal byproducts of bodily processes and have certain beneficial functions, increased levels of free radicals can permeate the tissues. Such permeation makes them detrimental to one's health. The products from free radical reactions are implicated in the progressive accumulation of changes over time, which in some individuals may eventually be recognized as disease. Free radical damage is now believed to be involved in a number of bodily disorders and diseases, including the two major causes of death, atherosclerosis (a leading precursor of heart disease and stroke) and cancer.[5]

We are exposed to significant sources of free radicals that exist in the environment. Two major environmental sources are the air pollutants nitrogen dioxide and ozone. They are of particular concern for individuals living in heavily polluted areas of the country, such as New York City, Los Angeles (the most air-polluted city in the United States), Boston, Baltimore, and Atlanta.

There are other sources of free radicals. Substances in cigarette smoke cause serious free radical damage in the lungs.

This not only happens to cigarette smokers themselves, but to other people who inhale residual smoke lingering in the air. Heavy metals and halogenated hydrocarbons, present in polluted air and water, cause free radical damage. Free radicals are also produced following exposure to ionizing radiation, as from an X-ray machine or from the atmosphere's concentrated cosmic and ultraviolet rays that bombard planes in flight.[6] Finally, there is growing evidence that essentially everyone in our society is exposed to free radicals, more now than ever before, because of the hole in the ozone layer. This is a layer of a special type of oxygen in the upper atmosphere that absorbs ultraviolet radiation. Without the ozone layer, more ultraviolet radiation reaches the Earth.

RESEARCH ON FREE RADICALS

Extensive research on free radicals and aging has been conducted at the University of Nebraska. Early studies by Emeritus Professor of the School of Medicine Denham Harman, M.D., Ph.D., the developer of the free radical theory of pathology, demonstrated that exposure of laboratory animals to radiation appeared to age the animals unusually fast. It caused an increase in free radical levels in their cells. Increasing the free radical activity in the animals was apparently speeding up the aging process.[7] Other research studies in animals and humans have shown an accumulation of free radical damage in the process of aging or during the development of degenerative diseases.[8–10]

To study the role of free radical reactions in cellular aging, investigators at Texas A&M University have monitored the effects of vitamin E deficiency in rats. They studied the appearance of a protein in red blood cell membranes that changes shape as the cell ages. Eventually, under normal conditions, the protein displays what is termed by the researchers as a "senescent cell antigen," an area of the protein that signals the immune system to destroy the cell. However, among the nutrient-deficient rats, red blood cells of all ages behaved like old red blood cells from control animals fed a nutritionally complete diet. The researchers concluded that nutritional deficiency, such as a lack of vitamin E, is the reason for premature aging of red blood cells, presumably because of damage by free radicals.[11]

Animal research has also documented the progressive accumulation of *lipofuscin*, or age pigment, as part of the aging process in every animal species studied. (Lipofuscin is what causes liver spots in humans.) This build-up of lipofuscin in cells over time is the most universal age-related change in cells. Lipofuscin pigments are thought to be the end products of free radical reactions in the body.[12]

ANTIOXIDANT DEFENSE SYSTEMS

Support for the free radical theory comes from research findings showing that a diet deficient in antioxidants—such as vitamins B, C, and E, and the minerals selenium, magnesium, and germanium—leads to the accumulation of a pigment similar to lipofuscin in a variety of tissues.[13] Evidence also suggests that animals deficient in vitamins and minerals are more susceptible to peroxide formation in body tissues.[14] Therefore, a deficiency in a vitamin such as alpha tocopherol (a form of vitamin E) may be a useful tool for evaluating the roles of free radical products in cell-membrane damage and the accumulation of age pigment in producing age-related changes in some tissues.[15]

There are defense systems to protect the body from free radical damage. These systems include both antioxidants and enzymes, substances that promote chemical changes within the body. Since their discovery in the early part of this century, vitamins have been accepted as major antioxidants in body tissues. For example, the antioxidant characteristic of vitamin E is considered to be a first line of defense against free radical damage.[16] The vitamin stops free radical chain reactions, inhibiting the production of additional free radicals, and confines damage to limited areas of the cell membranes.[17] Selenium, found in the enzyme glutathione peroxidase, is the second line of defense, and destroys free radical peroxides before they can damage cell membranes.[18]

Additional studies have shown that dietary supplementation with selenium and other antioxidants can significantly affect age-related changes in body tissues. Biological antioxidants, in particular vitamins A, C, and E, can inhibit the accumulation of damaging free radicals. Dietary vitamins and minerals appear to have a critical role in protecting tissues against the environmental free radical damage that usually is experienced in everyday living. Based on the free radical theory of aging, scientists believe that increasing the level of protective substances, including antioxidants, would tend to slow down the aging process and thus lead to an extension of an individual's normal life span.[19]

ANTIOXIDANTS IN OTHER ANIMAL STUDIES

The implications of various types of dietary fat on life span and age-related changes were evaluated in another study on rats. Results did not show differences in maximum life span between dietary groups. However, more rats fed a diet high in polyunsaturated fats and antioxidants were alive at a specific age than rats in all other groups. This beneficial effect was related to delayed onset and reduced incidence of cancerous tumors.[20]

Research at Tufts University on the effects of antioxidants in the brains of rats showed a protective effect of such nutrients as aged garlic extract, protomorphogens, spirulina, aspartates, ascorbates, glutathione, bioflavonoids and flavonols, oil of evening primrose, green barley essence, Siberian ginseng, niacin and niacinamide, vitamins C and E, zinc, selenium, germanium, and magnesium. (We'll take a closer look at these substances in Part II.)

The Tufts study showed that both diet and age had a significant effect on the concentrates of these nutrients in both the bloodstream and the brain tissue. Young and old rats were divided into two groups each. One group was fed a nutrient-poor diet. The other was fed a diet supplemented with antioxidants. After eight weeks, there was thirty-two times as much antioxidant in the blood of the supplement-fed young animals when compared with that of the nutritionally deficient animals, and three times as much antioxidants in the first group's brains. In the older rats, the supplement-fed animals had 1.8 times as much antioxidant in the blood and 1.5 times as much in the brain compared with the deficient rats. In old animals, relatively long-term supplementation (twenty weeks) was necessary to inhibit the formation of peroxides in the brain. The researchers concluded that antioxidant supplementation can play a major role in protection of the brain against free radical reactions and tissue damage.[21]

The researchers at Tufts University also conducted mouse studies on immune response and the aging process. They demonstrated that mice fed diets supplemented with vitamin E showed an increased immune response. The animal studies led investigators to conclude that increasing nutritional supplementation intake with age may retard the age-associated changes that lead to a decline in human immune system function. This decline in function makes us more susceptible to cancer and other degenerative diseases.[22]

HUMAN STUDIES: GUARDING AGAINST GROWING OLD TOO SOON

On the basis of animal study results, researchers believe that nutritional supplementation with a variety of substances may enhance immune response in later life among humans. They have conducted trials with adults over sixty years of age who took 800 international units (IU) vitamin E each day. The results showed that control of immune responses may become unbalanced as we age, and that nutritional supplements can reestablish that balance.[23]

A study was conducted among older people in Poland. The relationship between blood levels of vitamins and peroxides was investigated in 100 people between 60 and 100 years of age. After four months, average blood peroxide levels decreased 14 percent among those who took 200 IU of vitamin E a day, 8 percent among those who took 400 mil-

ligrams (mg) of vitamin C, and 20 percent among those who
took both vitamins. After a year, the blood peroxide level decreased 26 percent in the group receiving vitamin E, 13 percent in the group receiving vitamin C, and 25 percent in the
group receiving both vitamins C and E. The researchers concluded that administration of vitamins C and E, even at small
doses, caused a decreased accumulation of blood peroxide
levels in older people.[24]

Another experiment among older people was conducted in
Finland. It was designed to determine the effects of nutritional supplementation on mental well-being among nursing
home patients. The study evaluated the theory that a decline
in mental function is an early indicator of tissue aging, and
that antioxidant supplements inhibit accumulation of free radicals and lipofuscin. Fifteen older persons received daily supplements of 50 micrograms (mcg) of organic selenium, 8 mg
of sodium selenate (a selenium salt), and 600 IU of vitamin
E for one year. Study results demonstrated significant improvement in these people, as measured using a recognized
clinical assessment scale. Improvement was noted in the patients' general physical condition after only two months, and
their improvement continued throughout the study. The researchers concluded that their findings were directly related
to the action of vitamin E and selenium on tissue aging.[25]

THE ROLE OF ANTIOXIDANTS IN AGING

Death from free radical reactions—in the absence of injury or
overt disease—is most likely the result of a gradual accumulation of irreversible changes produced by these reactions.
Irreversible changes caused by free radical pathology slowly
impair function and eventually cause individuals to die before their maximum life span.[26] And virtually everyone is exposed, to a greater or lesser degree, to free radical reactions.[27]

Extending the length of life without enhancing the quality
of life is of little benefit. Evidence is accumulating from research results that long-term damage associated with free radicals can be controlled with adequate defense systems, espe-

cially through the use of antioxidant nutrients. These nutrients have a protective role in the aging process and tend to promote longevity. The important message is that use of specific nutritional supplements can help you achieve a longer, healthier, more vigorous, and generally better life.

Chapter 2

Stress as a Source of Premature Aging

Kenneth Greenspan, M.D., director of the Laboratory for Stress-Related Disorders at Columbia Presbyterian Medical Center in New York, once told a story about a fellow named Harry. Harry was under a lot of stress at work and at home. What was worse was that except for $30 in his pocket, only the $150 in his savings account stood between Harry and starvation.

One morning, Harry couldn't face his boss. So instead of going to his job, he went to a bar and wound up telling another customer his many troubles. Harry said, "You know, I need a vacation, a cruise maybe, and Greece is the only place where I feel I can unwind. Yet I have a total of only $180. Do you know of any bargain cruises?"

The man replied, "Relax. Go to the bank, withdraw all your money, and bring it here to me." When Harry returned, the man told him, "At 11 p.m. tonight a travel agent will meet you in the alley behind this bar."

That night, Harry followed his new friend's instructions and was hit over the head in the alley. When he woke up he found himself in the hold of a boat. He was sitting on a stool, chained to an oar that extended out through a porthole. A drummer sat in front of him, and a man with a whip stood behind. He was ordered to row each time he heard a drum beat. Any time he lost the beat, the whip cracked across Harry's back.

Harry rowed for weeks on end. Finally, he heard the captain on an upper deck telling the first-class passengers, "Ladies and gentlemen, in a moment we'll be landing at the Port of Athens, Greece." At this point, poor Harry turned to the fellow next to him and said, "You know, I've never been on a cruise like this before. Tell me, how much do you tip the drummer?"

CHAINED TO A LIFE OF STRESS

Just like Harry, many of us feel chained and entrapped by the pressures of life. We perform, and then judge our performance with the whip of hindsight. We then overtip the drummer of stress for the privilege of being on the bargain cruise. The external beat becomes internalized, and our own natural mind-body rhythms are censored out. We become totally focused on the external goal, and rationalize; after all, we are on our way to Greece, where we will finally relax.

Dr. Greenspan explains:

> Stress, the internal drummer, truly lies within us. So also does the solution to our human predicament. The answer is already there. We merely need to learn how to call it forth. . . . Think about an activity in which you experienced total relaxation and integration. It may have been a moment swimming, or making love, or dancing, or playing a musical instrument, or just quietly reading a book by a fire. Whatever else it was, it was a moment when you experienced an integrated peace and lack of stress. Now the issue is, how can you call forth the same response in your daily life?
>
> In most cases the answer is within ourselves. How can we find it? Well, that depends first on where we are right now. You can't plan a trip to Greece without a starting point, and you won't experience the arrival if you just row to the beat of an internalized drummer. Indeed, we must

first diminish the automatic stress response and then refocus so that we experience new options and response patterns.[1]

Scientists have been trying to understand how stress and its primitive response patterns can lead to chronic states of illness and anxiety. In this chapter, we'll first see how stress affects our bodies, and how our bodies try to adapt to stress. We'll then see how stress can be reduced.

THE PRIMITIVE HUMAN RESPONSE TO STRESS

Stress is a fact of life, from birth to death. As life grows more complex, stress becomes an increasingly pervasive and constant element of our culture. It reflects the pressures of life—both the ordinary pressures of day-to-day living and the extraordinary pressures that confront every person from time to time during life's struggles.

Of course, stress is not necessarily harmful. Some degree of stress is normal and is in fact necessary for daily functioning. Coping with an optimum level of stress keeps us mentally and physically alert and stable.

For early humans, the stress response was critically important to survival. In the face of physical danger, it served as an arousal mechanism and evoked a protective adaptation response that helped people fight the danger or flee from it. However, the primitive responses that were essential then are maladaptive today.

An understanding of the early human brain is fundamental to an understanding of our modern stress response. So is an understanding of the contrast between the chronic stress demands of our own modern culture and our biologically primitive response patterns, which evolved to allow for immediate survival under conditions of immediate physical danger.

What we define as stress today is the response to any demand of modern life that calls these primitive protective mechanisms into play. While each type of stressor—such as cold, heat, injury, frustration, joy, and so forth—has its own specific effects, all stressors possess the common feature of requiring adaptation. (For clues to a person's hidden stress response, see "Recognizing the Signs of Internal Stress.")

There are three different types of persons in terms of stress response:

- *Type As* are persons who externalize their stress by becoming visibly upset or engaging in aggressive behavior. They may eventually suffer from disorders such as ulcers, high blood pressure, heart attacks, and strokes.

- *Type Bs* are persons who internalize their stress. They may appear calm, but are inwardly tense and nervous. Their immune systems may malfunction, provoking serious conditions such as arthritis and cancer. They may also have family and job problems, and low resistance to colds and other minor infections.

- *Type Cs* are persons who cope with stress effectively, react to it calmly, and who know how to control their stress response.

STRESS AS AN OVERALL HEALTH PROBLEM

Stress becomes a problem when it overwhelms a person's ability to cope. For even the most stable person, daily bombardment by a rapid succession of events and changes may add up to an overload of stress. It is then that stress may cause adverse effects, both emotional and physiological. These effects can range all the way from mild emotional disturbances with no physical symptoms to severe emotional disturbance and crippling physical symptoms that often masquerade as organic disease.

Illness is also a major source of stress, and is in turn aggravated by stress. Stress has been implicated as a factor in more than 50 percent of all visits to physicians. Illnesses that have been linked to stress include high blood pressure, heart attack, tuberculosis, asthma, and ulcerative colitis.

Recognizing the Signs of Internal Stress

Can you tell when a person is trying to control a stress response? There are signs. If you have an opportunity to observe an outwardly calm participant in an emotionally charged meeting, watch that person closely. Neither the face nor the posture is likely to show emotion. Successful adaptation to civilization involves learning to hide one's emotions well.

Look closely though, and you may see at least two changes. First the jaw may be clenched, back teeth only. There may be no other change in expression. Second, the person may switch from breathing with the lower chest, in which the abdomen gently moves in and out, to more rapid upper chest breathing. That's because the abdominal muscles are tight when a person is under stress.

These signs clearly characterize the presence of stress patterns. However, there is another subtle change that you may not notice. This is the hyperactivity of disturbed organ systems in individuals with chronic disease. Disease is the ultimate sign of stress.

People differ greatly in their ability to cope with various stressors. The level or character of response to a particular stressful event or condition may vary greatly—and sometimes dramatically—from one person to another. This variation in response may be due to genetic predisposition, or to cultural, educational, or environmental differences. A stress that spurs one person to brilliant achievement may send another person to a psychological counselor of some sort, or to a physician with complaints of various physical ailments.

Diagnosis of stress-related illness is complicated. The patient rarely identifies stress itself as one of the problems that has brought him or her to the physician's office. Also, the physical manifestations of stress differ in each individual. When the person's problem is actually organic, the symptoms tend to be consistently related to a classic disease pattern or a specific body system. A pattern of many symptoms diffusely scattered through many body systems or organs alerts the physician to suspect stress as the prime cause of the patient's complaints.

THE GENERAL ADAPTATION SYNDROME

Biological adaptation to stress follows a definite pattern. The late Hans Selye, M.D., Ph.D., D.Sc., one of the great pioneers of medicine, developed a revolutionary concept of stress that opened new avenues of treatment. He discovered that hormones—chemicals that control various bodily processes—are a factor in the development of many degenerative diseases, including coronary thrombosis (blood clots in the arteries leading to the heart), brain hemorrhage, atherosclerosis (also called "hardening of the arteries"), high blood pressure and related kidney failure, arthritis, peptic ulcers, and cancer.

Dr. Selye labeled humankind's biological adaptation to stress as the *General Adaptation Syndrome*, which develops in three stages:

1. *Alarm,* when the typical signs of stress are observed.

2. *Resistance,* when the signs of stress disappear and the person adapts to the stressor. If the stress continues, adaptation eventually fails.

3. *Exhaustion,* when the initial symptoms reappear. If the stressor is not promptly removed, death ensues.

In looking at this syndrome, we see that a person's power to cope with life's demands is finite. Thus, all of us must learn to budget this fund of coping ability, or *adaptation energy,* as we do other limited funds, such as money and time.

Most people normally experience only the first two stages of this syndrome. However, stress can still cause diseases of adaptation, which happens when the mechanisms of stress resistance break down or go awry. High blood pressure, gastric ulcers, heart problems, and mental disturbances can all result from imbalances in body chemicals produced during periods of stress. Even when stress is not the primary cause of disease, it affects the course of every illness. Depending on age, diet, sex, heredity, previous sickness, emotional state, and many other factors, there is always one weak link that sooner or later cannot stand the strain and breaks down, causing a general collapse.

The successful management of humankind's limited capacity to adapt to life's demands seems to be synonymous with the very process of longevity and life itself. Dr. Selye had speculated that "aging may be an extended [general adaptation syndrome]." He added, "In any case, it is clear that the more we understand stress, the better we are able to deal with it. I am convinced that the achievement of a long and happy life depends on following a code of behavior based on natural laws and suggested by the discoveries related to stress."[2]

TWO APPROACHES TO STRESS-RELATED DISEASES

One might think that the consequences of stress have long been known. Quite the contrary. The medical concept of stress is of recent origin, and most of our knowledge of its emotional and physiological effects, and of the diagnosis and management of stress-related illness, has been gained since the 1960s.

Studies show that animals kept to a daily routine—being fed at regular intervals, living in moderate temperatures, and not being exposed to noise and flashing lights—live an unstressed life and age naturally. On the other hand, animals age very quickly when they are subjected to irregular feeding intervals, extreme temperature changes, and distracting noise and flashing lights.[3]

The same results occur in humans. People living in certain areas of the Amazon basin in Brazil, or the Hunza people in the Himalayas between India and Tibet, or the Vilcabambans located high in the Andes mountains of Ecuador enjoy a vigorous life of natural aging until they are well over 100 years old. People living in more modern societies, on the other hand, are exposed to stress from all directions and undergo accelerated aging. The difference between the two groups is not only in the degree and kind of stress experienced, but also in their resistance to such stress. Studies have shown that even in a stressed society there are ways to increase resistance to premature aging.[4]

There are two treatment approaches to stress-related diseases. One is the curative, or crisis medicine, approach. The other is the preventive, or lifestyle medicine, approach. The crisis medicine approach consists of treating the manifestations of stress—actual disease symptoms that signify the presence of ulcers, arthritis, high blood pressure, or some other severe problem. In contrast, the lifestyle medicine approach consists of directly addressing the actual cause of these diseases, namely the inability to cope with stress. One way of doing this is to increase the individual's resistance to stress.

A primary rule that governs our prescription for long life is that almost all diseases can be prevented. The way to prevent them is to realize that stress, or rather the inability to cope with stress, is at the root of most disorders. Stress education, an antistress diet and nutritional supplements, relaxation techniques, and physical activity—all play an important role.

Our philosophy is in harmony with that of the American Medical Association, which suggests that doctors put more emphasis on preventive medicine. Such an emphasis could help extend youth into old age and, by helping to prevent chronic diseases, build a healthier, more long-lived population.[5]

TECHNIQUES FOR OVERCOMING
EMOTIONAL AND MENTAL STRESS

Fortunately, along with knowledge of how stress harms the body has come the knowledge of a number of ways to combat stress. Such stress reduction methods do include pre-

scription drugs. But they also include many nondrug therapies, such as nutritional therapy, meditative breathing, mind
control techniques, yoga, and exercise. Additional methods include counseling, psychotherapy, relaxation techniques, biofeedback, and massage. These techniques are used to help a
distressed person learn how to alleviate stress through relaxation, accept the diagnosis that the symptoms are related to
stress and not to an organic disease, and gain insight into
the personal problems that are creating stress.

In most cases, the patient immediately responds to counseling and other nondrug therapy. Sometimes, it is necessary
to alleviate psychic and physical pain resulting from stress
with a tranquilizer before the patient can become amenable
to nondrug therapy. But drug treatment must be considered
merely a short-term, immediately useful method of alleviat-
ing the consequences of stress. The benzodiazepine tranquilizers, such as Valium and Librium, have become overused in
our society. They are dangerous when prescribed excessively
for quick alleviation of anxiety symptoms. Not infrequently,
these drugs cause side effects when taken too often.

A major problem of tranquilizer misuse grows out of insufficient public and professional understanding of the inter-
action of tranquilizers and alcohol—that is, the simultaneous
presence of a high intake of liquor with an excessive dose
of tranquilizer. Alcohol and tranquilizers don't mix at all. In
combination, *they can be lethal.* Both are addictive agents, and
when taken together the two drugs can result in depression
and anxiety, paranoiac-type mental illness, physical debilita-
tion, and possibly even suicide. Therefore, drugs must be
treated with great care.

Of the nondrug approaches, meditative breathing, biofeedback, and exercise are the most effective methods for reducing the stress response. Meditative breathing involves induc-
ing a regular, relaxed, slow pattern of breathing—with moving of the diaphragm rather than the upper chest. It immediately changes many of the physical indicators of the stress
response. For example, skin response to an electric stimulus
diminishes, while skin temperature rises, when you go into

a meditative trance. Breathing techniques are part of many effective forms of relaxation therapy.

Biofeedback is also a relaxation technique. However, it is more than that, since the equipment also teaches conscious control of some involuntary responses. Biofeedback teaches people how to alter their involuntary functions through use of a machine that produces a tone when changes in pulse, blood pressure, brain waves, or muscle contractions occur. Eventually, the patient learns to produce the desired changes without the machine.

Science has evidence that biofeedback may be helpful as part of an overall treatment plan for high blood pressure and cardiovascular disease. Biofeedback, along with relaxation and breathing techniques, is extremely helpful in the treatment of headaches, muscle tension, insomnia, and Raynaud's phenomenon, a condition in which blood-vessel spasms cause the extremities to become numb and cold.

It is important to remember, however, that relaxation techniques should not be overdone. More is not better. You can meditate for twenty to thirty minutes twice a day with no problem. But if there is an underlying depression or severe neurosis, meditating an hour and a half each day may result in psychosis. If meditation brings on symptoms such as anxiety, depression, or hallucinations, see your doctor right away. You may want to see your doctor before starting a program of meditation if you are prone to such problems.

A marvelously effective and currently popular nondrug therapy is exercise. Relaxation breathing before and after exercise can enhance its benefits. But you should also be warned against excessive exercise. People with potential heart problems may strain their heart muscles badly through the physical stress of exercise. After two to three months of breathing, relaxation, and biofeedback therapy, some people with cardiovascular problems have learned how to reduce the stress response so they can exercise without harm. Again, if you have any sort of serious medical condition, see your doctor before starting an exercise program.

THE ROLE OF STRESS REDUCTION IN AGING

We have seen how our ancestors' "fight or flight" response to immediate physical danger has led to our genetically programmed response to stress. Unfortunately, this response does more harm than good in the modern world, where stress tends to be more subtle—and more constant. As a result, a poor response to stress can cause physical changes that can, over time, lead to serious illness.

The good news is that we can learn to control our response to stress. Prescription drugs may help alleviate overwhelming anxiety, but only on a temporary basis. Stress reduction requires techniques such as meditation, biofeedback, and exercise that moderate our response to stress over the entire course of our lives. The purpose of these techniques is to improve one's behavior in response to pressure, or in response to the stress that pressure has evoked. Integration of these stress reduction methods into daily living, along with other healthy changes in lifestyle, increases the probability of living a long life.

Chapter 3

Brain Allergies and Premature Aging

She is only forty-eight years old, but, Helen C. of New York looks at least two decades older than she is. If seen with her twenty-year-old son, people sometimes think she is his grandmother. It's a sign that her physician's diagnosis is correct. Brain allergies have caused Helen to age at an accelerated pace.

For a long time, Helen has been aware that she reacts differently than other people to the environment around her. While others seem not to be affected by cigarette smoke in an enclosed area, for instance, Helen feels panic. The smell of perfume puts her in a trancelike state, and the odor of natural gas plunges her into schizophrenic behavior.

Eventually, Helen uncovered the source of her disabilities after consulting a physician who specializes in clinical ecology. Clinical ecologists investigate and treat conditions arising from alterations in nature. Armed with this knowledge, Helen took action against respiratory pollutants in her home, workplace, and other places. She avoids tobacco smoke, formaldehyde-impregnated wallboard, polyethylene carpeting and drapes, felt-tip pens, photocopy machine inks, computer-generated printouts, and other irritants. She has experienced improved health.[1]

Unfortunately, Helen is not alone in her disability. Brain allergies, and the accelerated aging they can cause, are not as uncommon as you might think. In this chapter, we will first look at the brain chemicals that can accelerate aging. We'll then look at the allergy treatments used by clinical ecologists, and how they differ from those employed by conventional allergists.

BRAIN CHEMICALS THAT ACCELERATE AGING

It would seem on first glance that allergies and aging are not at all related. However, it is not so puzzling once we realize that both conditions arise, at least in part, from chemical reactions within the brain. Science is only beginning to understand the numerous reactions that occur within the human brain, and how those reactions affect health. What makes the issue even more complicated is that allergies are related to addictions.

How are allergies and addictions connected? We first need to define our terms. *Allergy* is defined as a harmful reaction to generally harmless antigens, foreign substances that provoke a response by the body's immune system. The immune system is supposed to fight dangerous invaders, such as germs. However, it sometimes overreacts, and starts fighting invaders that are not dangerous, such as pollen and mold spores. An allergic response starts when a person is exposed to the allergic substance and develops antibodies against it. A subsequent exposure causes the release of irritating chemicals. More than 40 million Americans have allergic reactions to cigarette smoke, house dust, and pollens. Another 40 million people suffer from food allergies. Food allergies can be so severe that people have died after eating relatively small amounts of the offending substance.

Addiction is defined as a state in which the patient has a compulsion to take a specific substance, seems to require more and more of it over a span of time to satisfy the compulsion, and suffers withdrawal symptoms whenever the substance is withheld abruptly. In that respect some experts see behavioral similarities between addictions to narcotics, alcohol, and cigarettes, and, for some people, coffee, certain foods (such as potato chips), and, oddly enough, gasoline vapors.

Actually, allergies and addictions are different reactions to the same types of substances. A person may develop allergic symptoms to a substance such as tobacco: nausea, dizziness, coughing. However, that person may become addicted to the offending substance if exposed to it frequently enough. That's because frequent exposure suppresses the symptoms, which results in a state of relative relief from symptoms. This relief is conditional, though, because the symptoms reappear as withdrawal symptoms once the substance is removed. Thus, smokers smoke to stave off the symptoms of nicotine withdrawal because they are allergic to it. Unfortunately, the conditional relief of addiction is a source of constant stress.[2] And as we saw in Chapter 2, stress plays an important role in aging and illness.

Scientists believe that they know where in the brain these reactions take place. Among the billions of cells in the human brain, there is a cluster of only about 20,000 cells that appears as a tiny blue spot. This cluster, called the *locus ceruleus* (*ceruleus* means "blue" in Latin), is a center where anxiety, fear, and other emotions take shape. Many chemical reactions with wide-ranging effects take place there. For example, most of the brain's supply of norepinephrine, a chemical that increases blood pressure without affecting the heart's output, is made in cells of the locus ceruleus. Norepinephrine, which is produced when the body needs extra energy, is distributed to other cells in the brain through a complex network of nerve fibers. That such a small cluster of cells could have such profound effects is one of the locus's wonders.

The locus ceruleus is probably responsible for at least part of the drug-withdrawal process. Doctors who have studied the locus have come upon brain chemicals that accelerate aging, chemicals that may be related to brain allergies. According to Dr. Eugene Redmond at the Yale School of Medicine, these chemicals hold answers to the intricate problems of addiction, allergies, and aging.[3]

LABORATORY PROOF OF BRAIN ALLERGIES

Michael Russell, M.D., and his colleagues at the Brain-Behavior Research Center of the University of California, San Francisco, wanted to prove that animals could "learn" to be allergic to usually nonallergenic substances. They did this by sensitizing guinea pigs to a protein called BSA. Whenever the animals were exposed to BSA, the animals experienced what most people experience during an allergic attack: their bodies released histamine, a substance that mobilizes the immune system, into their bloodstreams. The more histamine that is released, the more severe the allergic symptoms.

Then came the crucial step. The researchers exposed the sensitized animals to BSA along with an unrelated odor—either a fishy or a sulfurous smell—so the animals would learn to associate the odor with the allergic response. Within weeks, the scientists found that the bodies of the guinea pigs were releasing histamine when only the odor was present, even though the odors used were incapable of causing a "real" allergic reaction. Like Pavlov's famous dogs, who learned to salivate when they heard a dinner bell, Dr. Russell's guinea pigs had learned to become allergic to things that supposedly could not cause allergies at all.

Dr. Russell believes the same thing happens to universal reactors like Helen C., people who react badly to tap water, plastic dishes, and other forms of the modern deluge of synthetic chemicals. These universal reactors seem to be allergic to the twentieth century itself.

"The point of our work is that it can happen to anybody," Dr. Russell says. "We're seeing more and more people who are developing allergies to everything from the smell of tar to ozone to any non-bottled water. . . . A number of these people are, in my view, behaviorally conditioned."

The work of Dr. Russell and his colleagues shows a new way the brain can trigger a measurable physical change in the body—in this case, through the immune system. Dr. Russell says that the cue for a brain allergy does not have to be an odor. Sometimes, the mere sight or sound of something associated with the first time a patient undergoes an allergic response may be enough to set off an attack in the future.

These cues probably are doing more to the immune system than just stimulating histamine release. Dr. Russell says that odor messages, for instance, go to the hypothalamus, a part of the brain that functions as a switching station between the nervous system and the rest of the body. The hypothalamus helps regulate everything from body temperature, heart rate, and glandular secretions to stress reactions, hunger, and thirst. How far learned responses will be shown to affect other bodily systems remains to be seen. Dr. Russell's guess is that if one immune system chemical can be behaviorally conditioned, there will be others that will react the same way. The immune system has generally been thought to be independent of the nervous system, and attempts to tie the two were seen as unscientific. We now know absolutely that both mental and physical well-being are vital for health.[4]

CLINICAL ECOLOGY VERSUS CONVENTIONAL ALLERGY TREATMENT

Clinical ecologists are doctors who believe that repeated exposures to various synthetic materials in our everyday environment contribute significantly to many medical problems. They treat some mental illnesses, for example, as allergies or hypersensitivities to one's surroundings. For the practitioner of clinical ecology, also known as environmental medicine, premature aging caused by allergic brain responses is a very real disability that needs to be treated and reversed.

On the other hand, conventional allergists maintain that only specified areas of the body can exhibit allergic reactions. They narrowly focus on asthma and hay fever, for example. These two health problems are well-accepted diseases to the conventional allergists. These doctors do not acknowledge that the brain, muscles, bladder, or blood vessels could be affected by a food item, electromagnetic energy, smoke, ink, contaminated water, or some other pollutant.

The clinical ecologists are considered "quacks" by their allergy specialist counterparts in conventional medicine. Thus, there are two distinct medical groups practicing allergy in the United States. This disagreement among doctors means there are two ways of dealing with allergies, only one of which is known to the general public.

Clinical ecologists have recognized health problems long before such problems have become generally acknowledged. For example, some people experience an adverse response to food in Chinese restaurants: tightness in the chest, headache, sometimes vomiting and upper abdominal discomfort. Scientists now refer to this collection of symptoms as the Chinese Restaurant Syndrome, which is caused by the food additive monosodium glutamate (MSG). MSG is a flavor enhancer that restores flavor lost in cooking.

The physicians who first warned the U.S. Food and Drug Administration about MSG belonged to the Society of Clinical Ecology (now called the American Academy of Environmental Medicine). This group, under the leadership of Lawrence D. Dickey, M.D., F.A.C.S., was the guiding force behind the 1969 decision by food manufacturers to remove MSG from baby foods because it affected infant nervous systems. (Despite the clinical ecologists' efforts, MSG remains virtually impossible to avoid in prepared foods, and in many spice-and-herb combinations. It is also still sold in supermarkets under the brand names Accent and Ajinomoto.)

Conventional allergists continue to contend that most common types of allergy must be mediated, or controlled, by an antibody called immunoglobulin E (IgE). IgE is concentrated in the lungs, the skin, and the mucous membranes. It provides the main defense against antigens from the environment. IgE reacts with certain antigens to release particular chemicals that cause reactions such as reddening of the skin.

Conventional allergists diagnose allergy based on results of the radio-allergo-sorbent test (RAST), which shows whether blood levels of IgE are elevated. RAST is of value when respiratory or food allergies are suspected. This test can alert a physician that blood levels of IgE are too high, and thus prevent a possible serious reaction when the patient undergoes skin testing. Clinical ecologists consider that most food and chemical sensitivities are not primarily mediated by IgE. They believe RAST should only be used to judge the severity of a food allergy.

Conventional allergists believe that the major allergens are dust, pollen, mold spores, and pet dander. They have declared in formal statements that foods rarely cause allergy other than those reactions that are anaphylactic in nature. (Anaplylactic allergies invoke severe, life-threatening reactions to foreign proteins or other materials.) As a result, conventional allergists think that patients with brain allergies are suffering from psychosomatic illness, or illness in which emotional problems are displayed through physical symptoms.

Most people do not know about the disagreement between conventional allergists and clinical ecologists. Because conventionalists control the editorial committees of medical journals, patient observations made by clinical ecologists have not been fully represented in the medical literature. That does not mean, however, that the clinical ecologists' view of allergy is not valid, or that clinical ecology cannot help bring relief from the symptoms that plague allergy patients.[5]

A NEW APPROACH TO ALLERGIES

Allergy plays a role in nearly everyone's life as the great imitator. It can produce symptoms in the brain that may send both patient and physician looking in the wrong direction for a diagnosis. If an individual has any evidence of respiratory allergy and simultaneously suffers from some type of dementia, a brain allergy should be suspected. An adverse response to a particular food, or to food chemicals and additives, is the most common cause.

Brain allergy causes swelling in the brain. This reduces the brain's blood supply, and so keeps the brain from functioning normally. A dysfunctional brain, such as one showing the presence of senility, causes the aging process to speed up.

There may be various signs and symptoms, such as physical agitation or lethargy, heightened or reduced alertness, and other symptoms. Additionally, brain allergy is a source of dyslexia, learning disability, and emotion problems, such as feelings of frustration, anger, anxiety, and failure.

Conventional allergists use drug therapy to treat their patients. Drugs may be used to treat allergy symptoms, such as the use of antihistamines to reduce the amount of nasal secretions produced during a hay fever attack. Drugs may also reduce the patient's sensitivity to the offending substance.

In contrast, clinical ecologists stress that the preferred treatment of an allergy is to eliminate its cause. They recommend dietary trials to find offending foods, and changes to make the home and work environments more allergy-free and ecologically sound. They emphasize that allergies can affect any area of the body, including the brain. This is because the substances that cause allergy, or that are released within the body during an allergic reaction, circulate throughout the whole system.

We are all affected by pollution. The damage it does shows up in a number of different ways, from physical signs such as wrinkles to mental signs such as negative attitudes. Pollution results in accelerated aging and shorter life. We have no armor against our surroundings, with the result that the majority of people suffer health problems of various kinds, both mental and physical. According to one source, between 60 and 70 percent of all symptoms that are diagnosed as psychosomatic are caused by responses to pollutants in air, water, and food.[6]

The irritants causing allergic reactions are often in our homes, which are sophisticated chemical environments. One in ten people living in industrialized Western countries, for instance, are allergic to the following pollutants: fumes from their heating systems, chlorinated tap water, cigarette smoke, chemical additives in foods, hair sprays, disinfectants and cleaning materials, wall paint, furniture polish, and floor wax, among others.

THE ROLE OF BRAIN ALLERGIES IN AGING

Our surroundings bombard us with a complex inventory of chemical pollutants. We are poisoned by and react to molds, fat-soluble products, dust, airborne contaminants, inhalants, artificial foodstuffs, petrochemicals, hydrocarbons, and more. Everyone is familiar with some of the respiratory allergy symptoms these irritants produce: a runny nose, watery eyes, itchy skin, sneezing, coughing. People are also familiar with some of the more obvious symptoms of food allergy, which can range from intestinal distress to, in extreme cases, death.

As we've seen, these irritants can also affect our brains, producing symptoms not generally associated with allergies, such as mental disturbances. Such brain allergies can also affect the rate at which we age. Not all doctors are aware of this allergen-brain connection. Therefore, the underlying causes of allergic responses are rarely identified correctly—if at all. This is why the patient must take action by seeking out appropriate medical advice and creating a personal environment that is as allergen-free as possible. He or she alone will reap the rewards of being released from the stigma of mental illness and the disability of old age.

Chapter 4

Hair Mineral Analysis and Premature Aging

One of the most common threats to human health around the globe is toxicity from heavy metals such as aluminum, mercury, and lead. The problem is greatest in industrialized countries such as the United States, Great Britain, France, Germany, and Denmark. To some extent, all drinking water supplies and nearly all food raised commercially are contaminated with toxic metals.

Through a great deal of research, it has been established that there are reliable relationships between the levels of minerals in the hair and those in the body's tissues. Thus, analysis of the hair's mineral content can provide a blueprint of mineral content in the rest of the body's tissues, including the heavy metal content. Such analysis can also show deficiencies in minerals that the body needs, such as calcium. Therefore, it is possible to read the mineral content blueprint and see where metabolic patterns are deviating from normal.[1] This is important, because heavy metals can accelerate the aging process, as can a deficiency in essential minerals.

In this chapter, we'll see how hair is analyzed and look at what the results might mean, including the presence of toxic heavy metals. We will then explore the causes of mineral imbalance.

WHAT HAIR MINERAL ANALYSIS REVEALS ABOUT BODILY PROCESSES

Blood, urine, saliva, and sweat tests all evaluate the body's liquid constituents. The vast majority of the body's functions take place not in the fluids, however, but inside the cells themselves. It is not part of standard medical testing to take cell samples, or biopsies, without a good reason for doing so. Therefore, an easy way to learn what is happening within the body is by evaluating the hair.

As far back as 1903, a French doctor named Ustis Matsuura reported that disease causes variations in the width of hairs. He noticed that a hair taken from an ill person is not as wide across as one taken from a healthy person. From his studies at the University of Strasbourg, Dr. Matsuura could estimate the duration of an illness and whether that illness was slight or severe.[2]

Hair mineral analysis serves to pinpoint the development of metabolic dysfunctions, or disruptions in the body's normal processes, before symptoms appear. While mineral imbalances in the body do eventually show up in the blood, they will not do so until the condition is so advanced that the individual is already suffering from overt symptoms. Tissue mineral analysis allows the physician to determine that an imbalance exists before that happens. The imbalance can then often be corrected through nutritional therapy.[3]

Traditionally, physicians have relied on blood analysis to find out what is happening within a patient's body. This is acceptable when the doctor needs to know the patient's response to stress, diet, and other factors. For elements such as heavy metals, however, the doctor needs to know how much of the substance has accumulated over time. In this case, blood analysis reveals little useful information. Hair analysis provides a better assessment of heavy metal concentration because short-term variations are averaged out. A hair sample is not affected by a meal eaten just before the hair is taken for testing, or by the patient's present stress levels.[4]

Still, certain external influences on the hair do affect the readings obtained through hair mineral analysis. While shampoos, sprays, and other environmental contaminants hardly influence test results, the chemicals used for bleaching, coloring, and perming can cause test results to be unreliable. If untreated head hair is not available, then pubic hair or nail (which is made up of the same materials) should be used.

We'll first see how hair mineral analysis is performed, and then see what the results of such an analysis may signify. (If you are interested in having your hair analyzed, see Appendix B for a list of testing laboratories.)

How Hair Is Analyzed

A hair sample is taken by cutting from two to four tablespoons of hair from the nape of the neck. The hair closest to the scalp is the newest growth and therefore supplies the most recent information on mineral usage within the body. This hair is also relatively free of airborne pollutants.

At the laboratory, the hair is washed with purifying chemicals and rinsed well with distilled water. This is done in order to remove all external contaminants that may disguise the true content of the hair sample without affecting the mineral content within the hair itself.

The technician then dries the hair, weighs it, liquefies it, and prepares it for testing. The liquefied hair is analyzed to determine how many parts per million or parts per billion of a specific mineral are in the sample. A computer is used to evaluate whether the level of that mineral is high, low, or normal in relation to all the other minerals in the patient's hair.

For example, a patient's analysis may indicate that a high amount of lead and calcium is present in the hair, in combination with a low amount of magnesium. The patient's doctor may then conclude that the patient is developing an arthritic syndrome. The doctor will probably prescribe magnesium. This mineral usually brings the high calcium down to the normal range and simultaneously prevents the lead from activating a chemical that destroys the lubricating fluid in the joints.[5]

The Significance of Minerals Found in Hair

Minerals are incorporated into hair, which is mostly made of protein, because they are needed to give structure to each individual hair. When hair thins because of illness, the size difference is due to a lack of concentration of certain minerals. The minerals incorporated into hair determine its thickness and color. For instance, grey or white hair generally contains fewer minerals than dark hair does.[6,7]

There are certain mineral deficiencies or excesses in a sick person's body, depending on the degree and length of the illness. Because hair is a depository for unused minerals, these deficiencies or excesses may be reflected in a hair analysis, which in turn reflects the mineral status of the body. For example, when radioactive minerals are given to a patient, as in a barium enema test for gastrointestinal X-rays, there is a surge of some of this barium into the hair. The same thing happens when isotope minerals, such as those derived from uranium and plutonium fission, are administered to somebody for diagnostic scanning purposes, such as a CAT scan.[8]

Therefore, hair may reflect excessive or deficient body levels of minerals as an early sign of disease. Mineral levels tend to change in everyone during an illness. Since hair grows a slight bit every day, each day's growth reflects the nutritional status of the body on that particular day, as long as external contamination is eliminated. When hair clippings are taken for analysis and the laboratory removes the external contaminants, a reasonably good picture of the trace element status of the period in which the hair grew can be determined.

Hair analysis can reveal two important things: the presence of heavy metals and the absence of important nutrients. Our foodstuffs often do not contain adequate supplies of certain minerals, such as calcium, magnesium, iron, copper, zinc, and manganese, and particularly vitamins, including B, C, and E. The human body requires these nutrients for many important purposes, one of which is to protect itself against toxic metal accumulation.

HEAVY METALS THAT APPEAR IN THE HAIR

Heavy metals are so named because their atoms are heavier than the atoms of other metals. They can also be called toxic minerals if present in the body in excessive amounts.

There are several common heavy metals, and they are common because they have many industrial uses. Aluminum, the most abundant metal in the Earth's crust, is not actually a heavy metal, although it is toxic. It, combines well with other metals. It resists corrosion well, and is used in paints, foils, welding, and high-tension lines. Arsenic, which can form strong poisons in combination with other chemicals, is used in the manufacture of transistor circuits. (For a famous example of arsenic poisoning, see "Hair Analysis Solves the Mystery of Napoleon's Death" on page 46.) Cadmium is used as an anticorrosion coating on steel and iron. Lead, one of the earliest known metals, is used in storage batteries and in antiradiation shielding. Lead poisoning used to be a problem in poor neighborhoods, where children would eat the sweet chips of peeling lead-based paint. Mercury, the only common metal that is liquid at room temperature, is incorporated into thermometers, electric switches, and lamps. In alloy form, it is used in dental fillings. Nickel gives alloys strength and corrosion resistance.

The associations between heavy metal exposure and various diseases, in particular those pathologies associated with premature aging, have been made over centuries. At first, specific occupations were tied to exposures to specific minerals: black lung among coal miners, arsenic toxicity among weed and tree sprayers, lead poisoning among automobile battery workers, and nickel dermatitis ("nickel itch") among electronics and computer industry workers. Mercury poisoning is thought to be responsible for suicides among dentists, who have the highest rate of suicide among the professional occupations.

Connections were then made between heavy metal exposure and other groups of people. Cadmium toxicity has been linked to premature death among cigarette smokers.

Hair Analysis Solves the Mystery of Napoleon's Death

The French Emperor Napoleon Bonaparte was exiled to the island of St. Helena after his 1815 defeat at Waterloo. He died there in 1821 at the age of fifty-one. A few months later, his death was officially ascribed to a "stomach disease," now recognized as a gastric ulcer. This was despite rumors of foul play that persisted long afterwards.

In the 1970s, an attempt was made to definitively settle the question of what killed Napoleon. Samples of his hair were analyzed for their mineral content. The investigators found that the emperor's hair contained about thirteen times as much arsenic as is normally found in someone's tissues. Thus, historians have concluded that Napoleon's death was probably due to arsenic poisoning, not stomach ulcers. They believe that either he committed suicide—he had tried to do so in 1814—or that he was murdered.

Alzheimer's disease has been attributed to aluminum exposure among elderly persons susceptible to aluminum toxicity.

Chronic poisoning from prolonged exposure to heavy metals invariably leads to pathology, progressive body system breakdown, and death. That is because these substances interfere with the feedback process that allows the body to function normally and keep itself in balance. This can disrupt the body's state of equilibrium, known as *homeostasis*.

On its own, the body does not ordinarily rid itself of metallic poisoning. Therefore, in some cases, heavy metal poisoning is irreversible. The body will eliminate heavy metals slowly, perhaps in six to eighteen months, if capable of doing so at all. Any attempt at detoxification requires the help of a physician using chelation therapy (see Chapter 13) and other detoxifying treatments.

Heavy metals must be removed from the body over a long period of time because distressing symptoms such as fatigue, joint pain, headaches, muscle aches, and gastric distress may accompany the elimination process. Such detoxification symptoms can also be counteracted by antidotes. For instance, if joint pain or excessive fatigue develops during lead or cadmium detoxification, the treatment is stopped for several days and lecithin capsules are administered.

Another reason that detoxification should proceed slowly is that a too-rapid release of heavy metals can cause serious damage. Lead released in excess, for instance, will be a burden on the kidneys and can cause damage. As another illustration, copper, a necessary mineral, can also be toxic in excessive amounts. It is normally stored in the liver. If this storage area is full, additional copper is stored in the brain. If copper is released too quickly, mental illness can result.

During detoxification, hair analysis is used to monitor how much metal is being removed from the body. Not all heavy metals stored in various parts of the body will show up on the first hair analysis. These undetected metals are likely to be so tightly bound to protein that they cannot be released until the body's chemistry changes enough to allow for their disposal.

Often, someone on a detoxifying program for heavy metals will see an increase in metallic levels on a follow-up hair analysis. What actually happens is that the patient's body begins to release excess metal from storage depots. It's an indication that the detoxification is working successfully.

CAUSES OF MINERAL IMBALANCE

Until recently, minerals have not been of much interest in medical circles. It was not until the 1980s, when it was recognized that osteoporosis could be corrected by the use of calcium supplements, that mineral nutrition gained a modicum of respectability. Now, more and more nutritional specialists believe that minerals are even more important than vitamins in the prevention and correction of premature aging.

It turns out that minerals are not only necessary for vitamins to function normally, but are necessary for activating or de-activating essential body catalysts called enzymes. Mineral im-balances can interfere with enzyme function. This in turn can interfere with the body's ability to repair itself, which can produce premature aging.

The importance of proper mineral balance can be seen in a number of examples.[9-13] Hair mineral analysis is useful in situations such as these:

- Although vitamin A is effective as a cancer preventative, its activity is greatly enhanced by the trace mineral zinc. Often, the failure of vitamin A to be effective is due to inadequate levels of zinc.

- A magnesium deficiency can be worsened by a high in-take of calcium because calcium counteracts magnesium, and vice versa.

- Sodium and vitamin E are incompatible. An individual with high sodium levels should temporarily stop taking supplemental vitamin E, or at least decrease the dosage.

- Zinc and copper are antagonistic to each other. A copper deficiency could be produced or worsened if zinc supple-ments are used when there is a low copper-to-zinc ratio in an individual's tissues.

- Vitamin C supplements act to depress blood copper lev-els in persons who already have low copper levels.

Improper diet is a source of mineral imbalance. Many peo-ple follow fad diets, usually for weight loss, that can disrupt their body chemistry and even cause harm. They may crave certain foods and eat them continuously with no regard to the effect those foods may have on their health. A craving may actually be an addiction due to an allergy to that food, and the allergy could worsen if the food is continually con-sumed. (For more information on the connection between al-lergies and addictions, see Chapter 3.) Food cravings increase as the allergies worsen. Excessive amounts of refined foods, such as sugars, refined flours, and other processed items, rob the body of nutrients, including minerals, eventually producing deficiencies and imbalances. Taking vitamin or mineral supplements without knowing what your specific needs are can often precipitate an imbalance that, in turn, can contribute to disease.

Most drugs also have an effect on an individual's mineral balance. Diuretics, for instance, must be coupled with potassium because they cause fluid loss and possible potassium depletion. Cortisone, given for inflammatory conditions such as arthritis, depletes the body reservoirs of calcium and magnesium. If continued for prolonged periods, cortisone can cause demineralization of bone and even bring on diabetes. It is known that both birth control pills and copper intrauterine devices (IUDs) can contribute to vitamin B_6 deficiency. Copper will then accumulate in the tissues, resulting in a zinc deficiency. Calcium may also build up in the tissues of women who use birth control pills.[14]

THE ROLE OF MINERAL IMBALANCES AND TOXICITY IN AGING

In this chapter, we have seen how the body's mineral levels are reflected in a person's hair, and thus how hair analysis can be used to determine the body's mineral balance. Hair analysis can reveal the presence of toxic heavy metals, such as lead and mercury. It can also reveal the presence of deficiencies in those minerals, such as calcium, that the body needs for peak efficiency, and the presence of imbalances among the essential minerals.

Both heavy metal toxicity and mineral imbalances can promote premature aging by interfering with the body's ability to repair itself and by upsetting the body's delicate internal balance. However, the effects of mineral toxicity or imbalance tend to occur over relatively long periods of time. Thus, hair analysis provides a way to determine a person's health in the long term.

Part II

Prescription for Long Life

As we've seen, our bodies have to battle many harmful conditions, such as stress and pollution, that can cause us to age prematurely. Sometimes, it feels like a losing battle. But it doesn't have to be. In this part, we will look at a number of ways we can fight back against the things that rob us of our youth. Some, such as fiber and yogurt, are well known. Others, such as OPC and Gerovital, are not. All of them can help us all fight the battle against premature aging.

Chapter 5

Minerals and Health—
The Major Minerals

Many people know how important vitamins are to proper health. However, most of those same people are just learning about the importance of minerals. Minerals may actually be more significant than vitamins for good health, disease resistance, and long life.

About 5 percent of the body's weight is made up of mineral matter. Minerals make up most of the structure of the bones, teeth, and cartilage. They are also vital for a number of bodily functions, such as good digestion, muscle movement, and the transmission of nerve impulses. Some minerals are called the major minerals because they are needed in relatively large amounts. Others are called trace elements, or micronutrients, because they are needed in very small amounts. For example, the Recommended Dietary Allowance (RDA) for calcium is 800 milligrams (mg), but the RDAs of many trace elements are so tiny that, in many cases, they have not been established.

In this chapter, we will see how minerals function in the body to help keep you young, and at some good food sources of minerals. We'll then look at the major minerals: calcium, phosphorus, and magnesium. For information on the trace minerals, see Chapter 6.

HOW MINERALS HELP KEEP YOU YOUNG

Minerals have a number of important functions in the body.
One of these functions is the regulation of bodily fluids. Minerals have the power to maintain the delicate internal water
balance needed for all mental and physical processes. They
do this through osmosis, in which areas with higher concentrations of minerals will always draw water from areas
with lower concentrations of minerals. (You can see osmosis
at work by putting salt on raw vegetables and watching the
water within the vegetables come to the surface.) In this way,
a balance is maintained between the fluid inside the cells and
the fluid outside the cells.

Fluid balance is important because our bodily fluids con-
sist of water and dissolved minerals, or salts. These mineral
salts, or *electrolytes*, generate tiny electrical charges called ions.
Each electrolyte is either positively or negatively charged.
Therefore, a cell is similar to a tiny electrical battery, with
both positive and negative poles. Good health depends on
the cell receiving the essential chemicals and minerals contained in this electrically charged fluid.[1]

Another function of minerals is to serve as catalysts, or
enablers, for vitamins. Vitamins are found in the greatest
quantities where increased amounts of minerals are present.
Plants bring minerals up from the soil in order to manufacture vitamins, and these plant minerals liberate the vitamins
in our bodies when we eat the plants.

The fact that minerals can enhance the function of vitamins has been shown in studies of patients. For example,
kelp, a seaweed, contains high concentrations of minerals and
vitamins (see page 56). When pregnant women took kelp, the
following benefits were reported:

- There was a marked decrease in the number and severity of cold symptoms.

- Capillaries, the tiny blood vessels that connect arteries to
  veins, became stronger. Thus, there was less skin bruising.

- The women were less fatigued.

- Women who had experienced arthritis symptoms noticed that stiffness and inflammation went away.

- Women who had eye problems, such as iritis and cataracts, saw those conditions improve to the point that treatment became unnecessary.

- The women were less constipated.

- The women reported improvements in facial complexion, as stated by friends and relatives.

- The quality and texture of the women's hair improved.

- The women's fingernails became less brittle.

- The women reported an increased sense of well-being.

Minerals serve a wide variety of functions:

- About 95 percent of the bones and teeth are composed of calcium, phosphorus, and eighteen other minerals. This requires an abundance of these minerals in the body's tissues.[2]

- Minerals influence muscular contraction and nerve response.

- Minerals are necessary for the creation of amino acids, the building blocks of protein.

- Certain substances needed for health require the presence of particular minerals. One example is hemoglobin, since hemoglobin production requires iron (see Chapter 6). Another example is the body's use of zinc in the creation of insulin, the substance that controls blood sugar (see Chapter 6).

- Blood clotting is controlled by mineral action. Thus, minerals must be present in order for wounds to heal.

- Minerals in the bloodstream act to create a germ-killing effect.

- The vagus nerve, which controls the digestive system, will not function without potassium.

- A number of minerals are required for alertness, energy, and mental function.

THE BEST SOURCES FOR MINERALS

The best sources for multiple minerals are brewer's yeast, alfalfa, sea salt, kelp, and cell salts. Fresh fruits and vegetables also contain healthy amounts of minerals, as does dried fruit. (For the best sources of some individual minerals, see the discussion of specific minerals in this chapter and in Chapter 6.)

As its name implies, *brewer's yeast* is used in the brewing process. It is a rich source of the B-complex vitamins, along with more than a dozen minerals. Because it is high in phosphorus, it should be taken with extra calcium (see page 57). Brewer's yeast is available in either powder or tablet form.

Alfalfa is grown as a source of hay. Its deep root system allows it to absorb a lot of minerals the mineral-rich subsoil. Thus, alfalfa has a very high mineral content. It also contains a number of vitamins, including A, C, E, and the B complex. It is available in liquid form.

Sea salt is obtained from sea water (most table salt is taken from underground mines). Sea water has a chemical composition similar to that of the body's liquids. This makes sea salt an excellent source of many minerals and other health-promoting substances.

Kelp is a seaweed that is readily available for use in the kitchen. It contains calcium (see page 57) and potassium, and a wealth of trace minerals (see Chapter 7). It also contains vitamins A, B_1, B_2, and B_3; pantothenic acid; choline; and various amino acids. Kelp can be taken in tablet, powder, or granulated form. It is especially flavorful sprinkled on steamed vegetables and salads, and can be used as a salt substitute.

Cell salts are tiny potent tablets that furnish concentrated amounts of twelve minerals, either singly or in combination. They can be purchased in health food stores.

When taking supplemental minerals, use the chelated variety for better intestinal absorption. The chelation makes it easier for the body to use the mineral. Chelated minerals are assimilated three times as well as ordinary minerals.

One does not need to eat as much protein when the body is sufficiently supplied with minerals in proper balance. Normally, 70 grams of protein are needed each day to sustain good health and longevity. When sufficient minerals are consumed, only 25 to 30 grams of protein are needed. This may explain why many vegetarians who eat an abundance of fresh fruits and vegetables, nuts, and grains enjoy long life despite the fact that they do not eat the recommended daily amount of protein. Fresh foods contain many more minerals than processed foods.

MAJOR MINERALS: THE MINERALS YOU NEED IN ABUNDANCE

The major minerals—calcium, phosphorus, and magnesium— are needed in relatively large amounts. It is a good idea to make sure you're getting enough of the major minerals before worrying about the trace minerals (see Chapter 6).

Calcium: Bone Builder and More

Calcium is the most abundant material in our bodies, and 99 percent of it is found in the bones and teeth. The other 1 percent circulates in the bloodstream. That tiny percentage can create problems for people whose bodies cannot use calcium properly. In these people, calcium can lead to clogged (atherosclerotic) arteries, which in turn can lead to cardiovascular and other diseases.

Calcium has many important functions in the body, not the least of which is helping to transport nerve impulses from one area to another. This function is tied to calcium's involvement in muscle contraction, including the contractions of the heart. Calcium's support of the nervous system also helps to keep a person in a calm frame of mind. When the blood calcium level drops, one becomes irritable and nervous.

Calcium works with protein and vitamin K in the coagulation of blood. It also is needed to keep a proper acid-alkali balance in the body and to displace strontium 90, which may be present in the tissues from radioactive fallout.

If calcium intake has been adequate, the body can draw from a special calcium storage space called *trabeculae* between the bones. The trabeculae are long, slender calcium crystals. They release calcium when an individual is under stress. If the person is deficient in calcium, stress will cause the body to pull calcium from the bones. This is a slow process, which may go unrecognized until osteoporosis appears. This condition, which most often appears in postmenopausal women, leaves bones thin and brittle.

Calcium deficiency symptoms include irritability, depression, nervousness, tooth decay, cramps (especially in the legs), insomnia, heart palpitations, retarded growth among children, soft bones, and brittle bones. When such a deficiency occurs, the bones do not lose calcium evenly. The jawbone shows the greatest loss, which results in inflamed and bleeding gums. Calcium is also lost from the spine and pelvic bones. The breaking of a hip or thighbone in older persons often happens when the bones having been robbed of so much calcium that they cannot continue to support the body's weight.

In order for calcium to function, other nutrients must be present. These nutrients include vitamins A, C, and D, and the minerals phosphorus and magnesium. These nutrients help in the absorption of calcium and, in turn, calcium aids them in their work. Calcium is the most difficult of all minerals for the body to assimilate and, like iron, requires an acid environment to make it available in solution for distribution throughout the body. If calcium is not properly assimilated, it can gather in tissues or joints as calcium deposits. This leads to such disturbances as arthritis, bursitis, and related conditions. These calcium deposits have been compared to the mineral deposits that build up inside a teakettle. Such deposits can only be cleaned with apple cider vinegar, which creates an acidic environment.[3]

Apple cider vinegar has been successfully used to treat arthritic symptoms of cattle. The virtues of diluted apple cider vinegar—just one teaspoonful to a glass of water—have also been extolled for human use. Vitamin C, also known as ascorbic acid, can also be taken together with calcium.

If calcium absorption is being hindered by a lack of hydrochloric acid in the stomach, hydrochloric acid tablets can be of help in the digestion of calcium, iron, and protein. However, these tablets *should not* be used by someone with ulcers.

Food sources of calcium include Swiss and cheddar cheeses, carob powder, collard and turnip greens, molasses, almonds, parsley, and Brazil nuts. If you want to use calcium supplements, take about 800 mg of chelated calcium a day in tablet or capsule form. You should not take calcium supplements if you have too much calcium in your body (a condition known as hypercalcemia) or if you have disease of the parathyroid glands, four small glands attached to the thyroid gland in the neck.

Phosphorus: Calcium's Partner

Phosphorus works in combination with calcium to build the skeletal system. Therefore, phosphorus is important in building strong bones and teeth. Approximately 66 percent of the phosphorus in food finds its way into the bones, while the remainder lodges in the soft tissues.

Phosphorus is a brain food. It forms links with fats and a chemical called lecithin to form phosphorized fats, the fats that are necessary to create brain cells. "Although 85 percent of your brain consists of water, the brain's solid grey matter is made up of phosphorized fats," according to nutrition author Carlson Wade.[4]

Phosphorus is necessary for the synthesis of protein, carbohydrate, and fat. It regulates the thickness of the blood, and works to neutralize excess acid in the blood. Phosphorus influences muscle tone and structure, and functions as a kind of accelerator control for the entire autonomic nervous system. This acceleration affects muscular contraction, gland secretions, nerve-impulse transfers, and kidney functioning. Phosphorus is also vital for cell reproduction and division.

Phosphorus deficiency shares many of the same symptoms with calcium deficiency: nervousness, osteoporosis, soft bones, deficient nerve and brain function, reduced sexual functioning, general fatigue, and, in extreme cases, irregular breathing and pale skin.

Natural food sources for phosphorus include cheese, milk, eggs, meats, raisins, mushrooms, wheat bread, oatmeal, walnuts, almonds, and rice. Because it is contained in many foods, there is almost never a deficiency in phosphorus.

When phosphorus is excreted from the body, it takes a certain amount of calcium with it. An excess of phosphorus can result in leg cramps, a sign of calcium deficiency. Therefore, calcium and phosphorus need to be balanced in a ratio of 2.5 to 1. Because lecithin, brewer's yeast, soda, and meats are especially high in phosphorus, extra calcium needs to be consumed when these foods are eaten in order to maintain balance. One-fourth cup of powdered calcium lactate or one-half cup calcium gluconate should be added to every pound of brewer's yeast. Vitamin D should be consumed with this mixture to help normalize the calcium-phosphorus ratio. As in the case of calcium, you should not take supplemental phosphorus if you have parathyroid disease.

Magnesium: Protection for the Heart and the Mind

Magnesium works hand in hand with calcium and phosphorus. It helps the body absorb calcium if enough phosphorus is present. However, if there is not enough phosphorus, magnesium can interfere with the body's use of calcium. Like calcium and phosphorus, magnesium is essential to healthy bones and teeth.

Magnesium is vital for preventing the onset of cardiovascular disease because it improves the tone of the muscles within the blood-vessel walls. This can help lower blood pressure in some people. Clogged heart arteries and heart pain respond to magnesium. Magnesium also helps the body rid itself of radioactive strontium 90, a component of fallout, and has found application as a kidney stone preventative. The mineral dramatically arrests the symptoms of neurological problems, such as those caused by polio.

Because magnesium is destroyed by the drinking of alcoholic beverages, heavy drinkers are helped by magnesium supplements. Magnesium's effectiveness as a natural tranquilizer gives us a clue to its use by the nervous system. Animals fed a magnesium-deficient diet overreact to even small noises. These symptoms disappear when sufficient magnesium is given to the animals.

Orthomolecular psychiatrist Abram Hoffer, M.D., Ph.D., uses magnesium to treat mental and emotional problems, such as irrational behavior. Hoffer even administers magnesium for serious mental problems, such as convulsions and insanity.[5] It has also been employed for tantrums, rages, epilepsy, and hand tremors.

Magnesium deficiency can lead to kidney damage and kidney stones, muscle cramps, atherosclerosis, heart attack, epileptic seizures, nervous irritability, marked depression and confusion, impaired protein metabolism, and premature wrinkles.

Food sources for magnesium are plentiful, and include lima beans, almonds, oatmeal, whole wheat flour, brown rice, all leafy vegetables, asparagus, figs, lemons, grapefruits, yellow corn, oil-rich nuts and seeds, wild rice, apples, soy products, unrefined vegetable oils, and celery. Raw food sources are recommended, as magnesium often is lost during food processing and cooking.

A good way to take magnesium as a cooling, nerve-relaxing beverage is to grind enough sunflower seeds to create tablespoon of sunflower meal. Next, place equal portions of beet greens, cucumbers, and cauliflower into a blender with the sunflower meal. Blend briefly.[6]

The RDA for magnesium is 350 mg. Because deficiency is common, a magnesium supplement is recommended. Take magnesium on a 1 to 1 ratio with calcium. Because of its alkalinity, supplemental magnesium should be taken between meals so that it does not interfere with the digestive process. Do not take magnesium supplements if you suffer from severe diarrhea or kidney failure.

In this chapter, we've discussed why minerals are as important as vitamins for good health. We've also discussed the major minerals, the ones that your body needs in relatively large amounts for optimum health. In the next chapter, we will discuss trace minerals. Trace minerals might not be needed in large amounts, but they are vital in the fight against premature aging.

Chapter 6

Minerals and Health— The Trace Minerals

In Chapter 5, we discussed some basic information on minerals and their importance to good health. We also said that the major minerals—calcium, phosphorus, and magnesium—are needed in relatively large amounts. Now it is time to discuss the trace minerals, or micronutrients, the ones that are needed in relatively small amounts.

The trace minerals include iron, zinc, copper, manganese, nickel, cobalt, molybdenum, selenium, chromium, iodine, fluorine, tin, silicon, vanadium, and lithium. New trace minerals are being discovered at a rate of two per decade. For example, the elements bromine, boron, rubidium, lithium, and strontium may also be essential in trace amounts. Even cadmium, an acknowledged highly toxic element, may be essential for growth in some animal species. (You should keep in mind that all minerals are toxic in overly large amounts.)

In this chapter, we will discuss four of the most important trace minerals: germanium, selenium, zinc, and iron. These minerals play many important roles in helping your body fight the effects of age.

GERMANIUM: THE IMMUNE SYSTEM BOOSTER

Germanium is one of the most exciting nutrients in the world of wholistic medicine. First used in Japan, germanium is available in this country as Germanium 132 (Ge-132, trademarked GeOxy-132).

While a complete set of studies on Ge-132 has not yet been done, it appears that this mineral has three main effects within the body. First, it seems to stimulate the immune system by stimulating the production of gamma interferon, a substance that has the ability to inhibit viral growth. It is not possible to produce large quantities of gamma interferon in animals and use them in humans, because the interferon produced by each animal only works in that specific animal. It is possible to artificially stimulate the human body to produce its own interferon, however, through the use of germanium supplements. Ge-132 can also stimulate the activity of another immune system component, the natural killer (NK) cells. Germanium's immune-stimulating properties make it useful in the treatment of chronic viral infections, including AIDS.

Ge-132's second effect, which is related to the first, is its ability to combat fungi. It may be especially useful in fighting the yeast syndrome produced by *Candida albicans*. This syndrome usually affects the skin or mucous membranes.

Ge-132's third effect is its ability to put more oxygen into the body's tissues. Many diseases are related to an insufficient supply of oxygen. Germanium acts as an oxygen carrier in the same way that the iron-based substance hemoglobin does (see page 69). People with Raynaud's phenomenon, in which blood flow to the extremities is reduced, may feel warmth in the affected fingers and toes thirty minutes after taking germanium. Healthy people can feel the warmth in a couple of minutes. Athletes taking it have noticed increased endurance.

Ge-132 has other functions. Parris M. Kidd, Ph.D., former director of the Germanium Institute of North America, writes, "Ge-132 has dramatic analgesic effects. . . . [It] apparently can enhance or substitute for morphine—reportedly 3–4 grams will eliminate pain of terminal cancer within 20 minutes."[1]

Dr. Kidd says that Ge-132 may normalize the blood's

chemical makeup, and that it can lower blood pressure without creating abnormally low blood pressure, even at higher doses. He says it also protects against the loss of bone among people with osteoporosis by normalizing the body's use of calcium.[2] It is useful in patients with elevated blood cholesterol levels.

Exactly how Ge-132 works within the body is not known, although there are several theories. One is that it shuttles oxygen into the red blood cells, which carry oxygen in the bloodstream, and then from the red cells into the tissues. Another says that Ge-132 acts within the mitochondria, the power plants found within all cells. Still another says that Ge-132 helps to remove hydrogen from the body, which aids the body in functioning normally.

Individual doctors have reported good results with Ge-132. Jeffrey Anderson, M.D. of Mill Valley, California, used Ge-132 to treat a 53-year-old man who had been suffering from recurrent diverticulitis, an intestinal inflammation, for five years. Anderson says, "He had almost a complete turnaround of all his symptoms within six to seven days. He was astounded and, of course, so was I."[3]

Germanium does exist in garlic and shiitake mushrooms, and in the herbs aloe vera, comfrey, and ginseng. (For more information on ginseng, see Chapter 14.) However, germanium is most effective when taken as a supplement. Ge-132 may be taken in capsule or liquid form. It could also be taken sublingually, in which a powder or dissolving tablet is placed under the tongue. A good general dosage would be about 75 to 100 mg a day. (See Appendix B for information on germanium.) It has been shown to be generally nontoxic, and no side effects have been reported. All traces of germanium are eliminated through the digestive tract within twenty to thirty hours.

SELENIUM: A FREE RADICAL QUENCHER

One essential trace mineral, selenium, deserves special attention because of its neutralizing effect on free radicals. As we saw in Chapter 1, free radicals are unstable molecules that are formed when the body processes oxygen. Free radicals also come from the environment. Air pollution, tobacco smoke, and pesticides all promote free radical formation.

To picture how free radicals affect the body, imagine a car traveling on a very crowded highway. Suddenly, one tire goes over a nail and blows out. The car swerves out of the driver's control, and crashes into another car. Other cars behind the accident cannot stop in time, and a multicar collision occurs. The cars in the accident represent molecules in our cells and the nail represents a free radical. That is how free radicals react with the molecules around them to cause cellular damage.

Selenium counteracts free radical damage in two ways. One, it helps chemicals within the body neutralize these unstable molecules, like a clean-up crew clearing a road of nails. Two, selenium can neutralize free radicals by itself. This makes selenium an antioxidant—a substance that fights against free radicals. Since free radicals are always present, the body needs a steady supply of selenium. Selenium acts in concert with vitamin E. In many cases, selenium neutralizes the same type of free radicals as vitamin E. (For information on other free radical fighters, see Chapters 7 and 9.)

Selenium is required for peak muscle tone and good muscle function. For instance, heart muscle that is deficient in selenium is flaccid and weak. Selenium deficiency has been linked to both heart disease and cancer. It is also required for pancreatic function.

One of Dr. Kurk's own patients has had good results with selenium and germanium. Sandra B., a homemaker in her late sixties, was experiencing itchy red skin blotches, headaches, constipation, allergies, depression, and a lack of energy. After taking the two minerals, and making changes in lifestyle and diet, Sandra found relief from her symptoms.

Selenium deficiency can be a problem because the soils in certain parts of the United States and Canada lack this mineral. This means that crops grown in such soils will not contain enough selenium.

Selenium is found in dairy products, seafood, wheat germ, Brazil nuts, apple cider vinegar, barley, whole wheat, bran, red Swiss chard, oats, broccoli, onions, garlic, molasses, liver, chicken, and brown rice. A good general dosage of supplemental selenium would be 200 micrograms (mcg) a day. Selenium has not been found to cause any side effects.

ZINC: THE ALL-AROUND AGE FIGHTER

About 2.5 grams of zinc are distributed throughout the body, with substantial concentrations in the eyes, kidneys, brain, liver, muscles, and male reproductive organs. It plays an important role in more than twenty chemical reactions. These reactions include:

- Detoxifying alcohol in the liver
- Helping the bones use phosphorus (see Chapter 5)
- Helping in the digestion and formation of protein
- Helping the body generate energy

Zinc is an important part of insulin activity, normal taste sensation, wound healing, vitamin A usage, and immune system activity. It also helps various molecules within the body retain their shapes.

There is evidence that a significant number of Americans do not get the proper amount of zinc. This evidence shows that marginal deficiencies are especially likely to occur among the elderly, children, pregnant and breastfeeding mothers, and the chronically ill. Members of these groups are at increased risk and should be monitored for zinc ingestion and absorption by their physicians and/or dietitians. Unfortunately, this is often overlooked.

Zinc deficiency can result in a number of different problems. Zinc is also an important part of male reproductive health. For example, it is a primary cause of impotence among men age forty-five and older because zinc is an important component of testosterone, the main male sex hor-

mone. Also, zinc combined with vitamin C is sometimes sufficient to counter the symptoms of chronic prostatitis, a
chronic irritation or low-grade infection of the prostate gland.

In several Midwestern nursing homes, women who took
medication for coronary heart disease had significantly low
zinc levels. Also, there was more zinc in the hair of women
in higher income brackets than in that of women from lower
income brackets. It was concluded that this difference reflected the different diets the two groups ate. (For information on hair mineral analysis, see Chapter 4.) Male residents
had problems with the sense of taste, problems that improved
after they received zinc supplements.

A zinc deficiency can also result in slow wound healing.
This includes superficial, everyday wounds such as cuts,
scratches, and insect bites, and serious wounds, such as broken bones, leg ulcers, and intestinal ulcers. Such problems
often improve when zinc intake is increased. Zinc is also beneficial when taken before and two to three months after
major surgery. Similarly, zinc should be taken by people who
have suffered major accidents or burns.

Zinc may be employed to treat eczema, a reddened, scaly,
cracking, itchy skin rash that often occurs in front of the el-
bows, behind the knees or ears, or on the wrists, hands, and
ankles. Eczema treatment should also include omega-3 oils,
and vitamins A, C, and E. Moreover, zinc can help reduce
the incidence of acne—better than treatment with antibiotics—
without encouraging overgrowth of the yeast *Candida albicans.*

Healthy adults require about 12.5 mg of zinc each day. The
average diet provides about 10 to 15 mg of zinc daily, one-
third to one-half of which is absorbed. There are several reasons why this mineral is not always absorbed. Zinc absorption is impaired when large amounts of calcium in the diet
bind with zinc and other substances in the intestines. Zinc,
cadmium, silver, and copper all compete for absorption sites
in the intestine. The zinc content of the blood declines with
increases in dietary fiber. Body stores of the mineral are not
readily mobilized, so a daily dietary supply is mandatory.

In general, animal foods are the best sources of zinc. Oysters are the best source by far, with 148.7 mg of zinc per every 100 grams of food. (The next best source, fresh ginger root, has 6.8 mg, and ground round steak has 5.6 mg.) The zinc in whole grains, even though it is not well absorbed, supplies a substantial contribution to the diet, especially for the vegetarian with a reduced protein intake. Most fruits and vegetables are poor sources of this mineral.

IRON: THE SUPREME OXYGEN CARRIER

Most people know they need iron for healthy blood. Iron is important to the blood because it is used to create a substance called heme. Heme combines with the protein globin to form *hemoglobin*, the oxygen-carrying chemical found in the red blood cells. Without adequate supplies of hemoglobin, the blood cannot carry as much oxygen as it should.

Heme also assists in creating myoglobin, a substance that serves as an oxygen reservoir within the muscle fibers. In addition, heme is used to build chemicals that fight free radicals (see Chapter 1). Small quantities of iron aid in other bodily functions, including nerve transmission, digestion, and blood clotting.

Iron is stored in the liver, spleen, and bone marrow. When iron supplies are low, these iron stores are expended first. Iron is carried through the bloodstream attached to blood lipids, or blood fats. If there is no more iron left in the storage areas, it is taken from the blood lipids.

Iron deficiency, or *anemia*, can cause a lack of heme in the body, which in turn leads to reduced hemoglobin production. A lack of hemoglobin produces the symptoms of oxygen starvation: weakness, fatigue, shortness of breath. A lack of iron in the blood lipids brings on signs and symptoms that include fatigue, headaches, heart palpitations, insomnia, loss of appetite, susceptibility to infection, sensory disorders of the hands and feet, hair disorders, a tendency to develop eczema, burning of the tongue, and pain on swallowing.

Sometimes, though, these symptoms may not appear. That can happen if a person has no breathing difficulties and thus is taking in adequate amounts of oxygen. When this occurs, it is called *masked anemia*.

Anemia affects the body's production of heat. One study showed that iron-deficient women do not tolerate cold very well, and that iron supplementation improves cold tolerance.[4] Women are especially prone to iron deficiency because blood levels of iron for women are known to decrease during menstruation. However, elevated iron levels can result from the use of birth control pills.

Iron deficiency is the number-one deficiency disease affecting the populations of industrialized western nations, as confirmed by studies in Great Britain, the United States, Switzerland, Sweden, and Germany. The recommended daily allowance for iron is 18 mg per day. The American diet provides about 6 mg of iron per 1,000 calories. The average American eats about 3,000 calories a day, which does result in an iron intake of about 18 mg. However, hardly more than 1 mg of that 18 mg is utilized by the body. (In contrast, the Bantu of South Africa consume about 100 mg per day because their dietary staples, porridge and kaffir beer, are both prepared in iron pots.)

Our bodies cannot readily use the type of iron found in food because much of it is chemically unabsorbable—the average absorption rate is only about 2 to 5 percent. The iron in food must be acted on by the digestive system and reduced to a form suitable for absorption, and a number of factors can interfere with this process. Absorption can be limited in individuals with food allergies, or by the intake of too much phosphate (such as by drinking excessive soda). Coffee or tea consumed with a meal or one hour after a meal significantly inhibits the absorption of dietary iron. Americans tend to eat foods with a low iron content, such as milk and refined carbohydrates. Iron absorption can also be affected by a low gastric acid level, gastrointestinal surgery, protracted bouts of diarrhea, and both prescription and over-the-counter antacid drugs.

Supplementation is needed. According to one study, "Anyone in the fifth decade of life and older should be supplementing with iron."[5] Iron supplements are often included in multivitamin/mulitmineral tablets. Iron can also be taken in liquid form. However, there are conditions under which too much iron can build up in the body. One is a rare disease called hemochromatosis, which is marked by bronze skin pigmentation, diabetes, and heart and liver problems. Excess iron can also cause other problems. For this reason, iron supplements should only be taken under a doctor's supervision.

As we've seen, minerals perform important functions throughout the body. But minerals are just the first part of the long-life prescription. In the next chapter, we'll look at a nutrient called coenzyme Q_{10} that can help your heart stay healthy.

Chapter 7

Stopping the
Free Radical Attack
With Vitamins and Coenzyme Q_{10}

We have discussed how unstable compounds called free radicals can damage our cells through a process called oxidation (see Chapters 1 and 6). As we've said, free radicals are not only produced by our own bodies, but also by various sources in the environment. There are thousands of environmental poisons that contain a number of free radical compounds. The damage caused by free radicals accumulates over time, and speeds up the aging process.

However, we have also seen how substances called antioxidants can help keep us young by neutralizing free radicals and limiting cell damage. Some vitamins, such as beta-carotene and vitamin E, are well-known antioxidants. So is selenium, a mineral we discussed in Chapter 6. But vitamins and minerals are not the only antioxidants. One of the most exciting discoveries in recent years has been a potent free-radical fighter called coenzyme Q_{10} (CoQ), a substance that can help strengthen the heart. CoQ, when taken as part of an overall treatment plan, can help heart patients live longer, healthier lives.

In this chapter, we'll see how environmental free radicals attack our bodies, and how antioxidants fight back. We'll then discuss CoQ—what it is, how it works in the body, and its potential benefits, especially its powerful effect on cardiovascular health.

ENVIRONMENTAL FREE RADICALS AND AGING

Environmental toxins are everywhere. They come from a variety of sources, including industrial waste, engine exhaust, and residential refuse. For older people, such pollutants and the diseases associated with them can lead to premature aging and its associated diseases. For example, environmental toxins are largely responsible for the high rates of eye diseases such as cataracts, glaucoma, and macular degeneration experienced by older people.[1]

Air pollution is one of the worst offenders, and ozone and nitrogen dioxide are two of the worst air pollutants. Ozone markedly increases a person's susceptibility to respiratory diseases and reduces lung capacity.[2] Tobacco smoke is a significant source of nitrogen dioxide. In fact, sidestream smoke—the smoke that people other than the smoker are exposed to—contains higher concentrations of potentially dangerous pollutants than does the mainstream smoke inhaled by the smoker. That is because sidestream smoke does not pass through the cigarette filter.

Nitrogen dioxide and ozone generate potent free radicals that can damage the eyes and lungs. Since the eyes and lungs are the primary targets for airborne free radicals, those organs must depend on particularly effective antioxidant defense mechanisms for protection against disease.

Vitamins are the mainline defense against premature aging and the bodily deterioration that results from exposure to airborne free radicals. Important antioxidant vitamins include the full B-complex group, vitamin E, vitamin C, and vitamin A (and vitamin A's precursor, beta-carotene). These vital substances influence the lung's susceptibility to free radicals in inhaled pollutants. (For dosage amounts, see Chapter 18.) Many of these antioxidant vitamins have also shown an ability to protect the body against free-radical eye damage. In both organs, antioxidants can reduce the risk of cellular abnormalities caused by free radicals. Such abnormalities can result in disease, including lung cancer, oral cancers, asthma, cataracts, and vision loss.

CoQ works in tandem with the antioxidant vitamins to help prevent degenerative diseases. For example, atmospheric oxygen diffuses directly into the eye through the cornea, the tissue that covers the front of the eye. Free radicals tend to diffuse into the eye along with the oxygen, and light-induced free radical damage can contribute to cataracts. However, the combination of CoQ, vitamin E, vitamin C, vitamin A, and beta-carotene may protect eye tissues against cataract formation in later life.[3-6]

COENZYME Q₁₀: FREE RADICAL QUENCHER

Coenzyme Q_{10} was first extracted in its pure form from beef heart muscle by scientists at the University of Wisconsin. It is a vitaminlike substance that is also called ubiquinone because it is ubiquitously present throughout the human body. (Nutritional chemists know of ten different coenzyme Qs, but only the tenth one has been found extensively in the humans.)

CoQ is found in all organs, but most abundantly in those organs that require a large supply of energy, such as the stomach, intestines, heart, liver, uterus, and testicles. It is also found in large amounts in the immune system. CoQ acts as a catalyst, or an enabler, in the chain of chemical reactions that allows the body's cells to create energy. A lack of CoQ is believed to be a factor in the aging process, since levels of the compound decrease as a person ages.

CoQ is known to quench free radicals because of its antioxidant effect. The compound strengthens cell membranes, which are easily damaged by free radicals. Although not itself classified as a vitamin, CoQ behaves in a manner similar to that of vitamin E. Moreover, clinical studies show that it aids in lowering elevated blood pressure, benefits those with gum disease, reduces symptoms in people with diabetes and allergies, and helps correct impaired immunity conditions.[7-14] Other reports indicate that CoQ is useful for treating muscular dystrophy and other muscle diseases. An editorial in one medical journal says, "CoEnzyme Q_{10} is the only known substance that offers a safe and improved quality of life for . . . patients [with] muscle disease."[15]

CoQ's role in energy productions means that it can benefit people who suffer from fatigue. This includes the fatigue associated with Epstein-Barr syndrome. More energy production means that more calories are burned. Therefore, CoQ can be used, along with dietary controls, in the treatment of obesity. CoQ can also be taken by athletes to enhance athletic performance.[16]

CoQ tends to protect heart tissue from the effects of Adriamycin, a cancer chemotherapy drug that is highly toxic to the heart.[17,18] Unfortunately, the conventional medical community has mostly ignored CoQ as a way of offsetting cardiac side effects in patients who are undergoing Adriamycin treatment.

CoQ AS A TREATMENT FOR HEART DISEASE

CoQ is a major advance in the treatment of heart failure. It has proven itself useful in treating various types of heart problems, including:

- Congestive heart failure, in which the heart cannot properly circulate blood throughout the body. This leads to breathing difficulties and swollen ankles

- Arrhythmia, or irregular heartbeat

- Angina pectoris, or pain caused by a reduced amount of oxygen reaching the heart

CoQ helps the heart because it increases energy production within the heart muscle. This allows the heart to utilize the nutrients and oxygen it receives more efficiently. CoQ also improves the heart's pumping action and electrical activity, which allows the heart to do more work with each beat, and to beat on a steady, rhythmic basis.

CoQ's effectiveness has been demonstrated in a number of

studies. In one study, twelve people with stable angina pectoris received 150 mg of either CoQ or a placebo (an inert pill) daily. After four weeks, the patients who received CoQ experienced a 53 percent reduction in the frequency of angina-pain episodes. These patients were also better able to tolerate exercise, as shown by the fact that their average treadmill tolerance time increased from 345 seconds to 406 seconds.[19]

In a study of 80 patients, daily dosages of CoQ for twelve weeks significantly increased the heart's pumping action and reduced shortness of breath. In addition, 89 percent of the patients experienced increased muscle strength.[20]

Twelve patients with advanced congestive heart failure did not respond well to diuretics and digitalis, the standard drugs prescribed for heart failure. These patients received 100 mg of CoQ daily and were followed for seven months. The patients reported that they felt less tired. Their activity tolerance increased, and their shortness of breath at rest disappeared. They also experienced a decrease in heart rate, a sign of increasing heart strength.[21]

Thirty-four patients with severe congestive heart failure and heart enlargement received 100 mg of CoQ daily. Of these people, 82 percent improved, as shown by enhanced pumping action and increases in the amount of blood pumped with each heartbeat. Two-year survival rate was 62 percent, compared with 25 percent for a similar series of patients treated by conventional methods alone.[22]

Several studies indicate that CoQ improves symptoms in arrhythmia patients, including those who experience arrhythmia as a side effect of drugs that affect mental functioning.[23,24]

In Japan, CoQ has been employed for several decades to treat cardiac disease as part of an overall treatment program for heart disease. Japanese clinical research shows that about 70 percent of patients with congestive heart failure benefit from administration of the compound.[25] In 1982 alone, about seven million cardiac patients in Japan were treated with CoQ, and that number has been growing each year.

Despite this record, American and European cardiologists have not accepted CoQ as an adjunctive treatment for heart disease. The problem—as with most nutritional therapies—has been the absence of a monitoring technique acceptable to the U.S. Food and Drug Administration that could prove the effectiveness of CoQ.

Evidence of CoQ's effectiveness now exists. Karl Folkers, Ph.D., former director of the Institute for Biomedical Research at the University of Texas, had been studying CoQ since the 1950s. With colleagues at the Scott and White Clinic in Temple, Texas, and Methodist Hospital in Indianapolis, Dr. Folkers found that CoQ can help both healthy people and patients with advanced heart disease. The response of the heart disease patients is often spectacular, and there are no side effects.[26]

PROPER DOSAGES OF CoQ

CoQ can be found in several foods, including beef heart; salmon, mackerel, sardines, and other cold-water fish; peanuts; and spinach. However, it is most easily taken in supplemental tablets or capsules of 10 mg, 20 mg, and 30 mg. Some clinical trials have used as much as 600 mg a day, but most studies have reported on patients receiving 50 to 300 mg daily.

We suggest that you look for a brand name when you buy CoQ, since not all products contain this substance in its purest form. It should be bright yellow, and the powdered form should have very little taste. Store it away from heat and light, since heat can cause CoQ to deteriorate.

Table 7.1 gives suggested amounts of CoQ for different conditions. Anyone with a pre-existing medical condition should *always* talk to his or her doctor before starting any supplement program. It is especially important that a doctor monitor the usage of dosages greater than 30 mg in heart patients, because stopping and starting CoQ therapy *could result in a relapse.* (Patients show improvement when they resume taking CoQ.) Remember, CoQ should always be used as part of an overall treatment program, in addition to other forms of therapy.

Table 7.1. Suggested CoQ Dosages

Condition	Dosage
Ischemic heart disease Chronic stable angina pectoris Decreased cardiac output Cardiomyopathies Congestive heart failure Cerebral vascular disease Essential high blood pressure Viral myocarditis Cardiac arrhythmias	100 mg to 150 mg daily in a divided dose (the average dose being 100 mg). In acute conditions, 300 mg in a divided dose for the first three days.
Muscular dystrophies Neurogenic atrophies	100 mg daily in divided doses. Some people will initially require 250 mg to 1 gm daily.
Allergy Epstein-Barr syndrome* Enhancement of immune response Chronic periodontal disease	80 mg to 150 mg daily in divided doses.
Obesity Sports medicine Fatigue	30 mg to 50 mg twice daily.

*Some patients with chronic Epstein-Barr infection may require dosages of 150 to 300 mg initially, along with additional nutrients: L-carnitine, 500 to 750 mg twice daily; biotin, 10 to 20 mg daily; selenium, 200 to 400 mcg daily.

The side effects of CoQ supplementation are minimal. Even high dosages generally do not bring on the potential common side effects such as gastrointestinal upset, loss of appetite, nausea, and diarrhea.

CoQ supplementation is a good idea for anyone who has reached middle age. It can help prevent a number of health problems that eventually afflict older individuals. However, CoQ's greatest benefit is for heart patients. Patients with the severest forms of cardiac disease should take CoQ as a lifetime therapy. In the next chapter, we'll look at niacin, another heart-healthy substance.

Chapter 8

Niacin—A Vitamin for Long Life

O ne of the most important ways to keep old age at bay is to keep your heart healthy. In Chapter 7, we discussed a little-known nutrient called coenzyme Q_{10}, and how it can benefit people with heart disease. In this chapter, we'll discuss a well-known nutrient called niacin, and how it too is important to heart health.

Niacin (vitamin B_3) is part of the B-complex group of vitamins. These substances are used throughout the body in dozens of different ways. They play vital roles in nervous system function, and therefore alleviate symptoms such as anxiety and mild depression. They also support the immune system and protect the body from the effects of stress.

The B vitamins play important roles in the circulatory system, and one of the most vital of these roles is played by niacin. In this chapter, we'll see how niacin works within the body and how it keeps the heart healthy, especially when paired with the mineral chromium.

HOW NIACIN WORKS IN THE BODY

Of all the nutrients, niacin was one of the first to be used as a medicinal supplement. In 1913, niacin, then called nicotinic acid, was isolated for the first time from rice polishings.

In 1931, researchers found that both the red blood cells and the heart muscle contained nicotinic acid. Verification of its value in human nutrition led researchers to conclude that it was an essential dietary ingredient. In 1937, niacin was identified as the third B vitamin. Shortly thereafter, scientists said that niacin was effective in treating pellagra, a deficiency disease that had afflicted thousands of people in the southern United States.[1]

Most of the niacin in our bodies is taken directly from the food we eat. However, an amino acid, or protein building block, called tryptophan can be converted to niacin in the presence of pyridoxine (vitamin B_6). In humans, approximately 60 mg of tryptophan produces 1 mg of niacin.[2] Therefore, it is vital to eat enough protein, containing adequate amounts of tryptophan, to avoid niacin deficiency. It is also important to maintain a good intake of the other B vitamins and of vitamin C, because these substances are required for the easy conversion of tryptophan to niacin.

Once niacin is absorbed into the bloodstream, it is incorporated into a substance called niacinamide. Niacinamide is a coenzyme, a substance that helps promote chemical reactions within the body. More than forty biochemical reactions depend on this coenzyme, and they all involve assisting the cells to generate energy. Niacinamide also helps the body use fats and proteins.

Supplemental niacin produces an initial drop in levels of blood fats, possibly by keeping fats from moving out of the body's fat-storage tissue.[3] Supplemental niacin also reduces levels of triglycerides, the most common form of fat within the body, and the levels of cholesterol found in low density (LDL) and very low density (VLDL) lipoproteins.[4] LDL is popularly known as "bad cholesterol," for good reason—it is the form of cholesterol that gathers in deposits on the inside of the blood vessels. When this process, called atherosclerosis, occurs in the blood vessels that feed the heart, it is called coronary artery disease. This can lead to chest pains called angina pectoris, in which the heart cannot get all the oxygen it needs. Atherosclerosis may lead to a heart attack, in which a clot becomes stuck in one of the narrowed, stiffened arteries and shuts down blood flow to a portion of the heart muscle. Therefore, by reducing the amount of LDL cholesterol in the blood, niacin can help prevent heart disease.

On the other hand, high density lipoprotein (HDL) is known as "good cholesterol" for its ability to remove LDL from the bloodstream. Niacin tends to increase levels of HDL in the blood, and keeps the blood from becoming too sticky, which can help prevent the formation of dangerous blood clots. And the vitamin stimulates the formation of substances called prostaglandins, which help keep the blood vessels healthy.

When people are given niacin intravenously, there is an increase in blood flow to both the skin of the hands and the muscle of the forearms.[5] There is no change in blood pressure during these niacin infusions, although there is a moderate increase in pulse rate. Consequently, the intravenous infusion of niacin is an excellent treatment for patients who have arterial blockages in the limbs, such as patients with peripheral vascular disease.

NIACIN SUPPLEMENTS AND THE CHROMIUM CONNECTION

There is no doubt as to niacin's beneficial effects on the heart. However, niacin supplements are available in different forms, each of which has a very different effect on the body. One of the most prominent effects of niacin is a sunburn-like flushing of the face and neck. This niacin flush happens when tiny blood vessels in the skin relax, allowing more blood to flow into the skin.[6] The flushing occurs about fifteen minutes after the niacin is taken and lasts for about a half hour. Supplements that are in the form of niacinamide do not produce this flush. However, it is believed that niacin reduces cholesterol levels when it is converted to niacinamide in the liver. Therefore, niacinamide supplements do not reduce cholesterol levels.

When plain supplemental niacin is taken, blood niacin lev-

els reach a peak in fifteen to thirty minutes, and then rapidly decline.[7] Therefore, many manufacturers of nutritional supplements have developed special time-release forms of niacin.
These forms provide a more consistent release of niacin into
the bloodstream with a reduced niacin flush.

Many physicians have preferred time-release forms of
niacin because of the reduced flush and reductions in other
side effects. Such side effects include itching, skin rash, nausea, diarrhea, and blurred vision. Time-release niacin is also
less likely to aggravate pre-existing conditions, such as peptic ulcers, gout, liver damage, and heart arrhythmia.

However, some doctors now think that *time-release niacin
may cause liver damage* at lower doses than regular niacin, and
in a much shorter period of time. High doses of niacin have
caused liver damage in people who took sustained-release
niacin purchased without a prescription. Therefore, we do *not*
recommend time-release niacin.

There is also evidence that niacin can aggravate diabetes
and may even induce the disease in borderline diabetics. Diabetes occurs when the body can no longer control the
amount of glucose, or blood sugar, in the bloodstream. The
disease can take one of two forms. In insulin-dependent diabetes mellitus (IDDM), the body's own immune system attacks cells in the pancreas that make insulin, the chemical
that controls blood glucose levels. This can eventually result
in the complete loss of insulin. The patient then needs to
self-administer insulin injections. In non-insulin-dependent diabetes mellitus (NIDDM), the body produces insulin, but the
insulin becomes less effective over time. Eventually, there is
both too much glucose and too much insulin in the bloodstream. The patient then needs to control glucose and insulin
levels through a combination of diet and drugs.

Researchers from the University of Texas Southwestern
Medical Center in Dallas studied the use of niacin therapy
in thirteen NIDDM patients. The niacin did reduce total cholesterol levels by 24 percent and did increase HDL levels by
34 percent; however, niacin significantly lessened the body's
ability to control blood sugar. The study's authors, Abhimany

Garg, M.D., and Scott M. Grundy, Ph.D., warn that niacin
. . . may turn some people into diabetics, especially people
with elevated triglyceride levels."[8] This is a cause for concern,
since NIDDM patients are two to three times more likely to
have high triglyceride levels than nondiabetics.

The University of Texas study also showed that the use of
supplemental niacin led to increased levels of uric acid in the
blood, a problem that usually leads to gouty arthritis even
in nondiabetic individuals. In this condition, uric acid crystals gather in the joints, especially that of the big toe, producing severe pain. Since diabetics are predisposed to gout,
niacin increased this tendency.

How can you take niacin for your heart without suffering
such side effects? The key seems to be the trace mineral
chromium. (For information on minerals, see Chapters 5 and
6.) Combining chromium and niacin in a form called chromium polynicotinate allows much smaller amounts of niacin to
be taken. This results in significantly lower blood levels of
cholesterol with fewer side effects. The use of chromium
polynicotinate also prevents a possible chromium deficiency.
Researchers have found that most people do not obtain
enough chromium in their diets.[9–11]

Doctors have used chromium and niacin together to reduce
blood cholesterol levels. Martin Urberg, M.D., of Wayne State
University School of Medicine in Michigan, gave a combination of 200 mcg of chromium and only 100 mg of niacin a
day to two patients. These patients saw their levels of LDL
cholesterol decrease by 23 percent and 30 percent.[12] Even
though it only involved two patients, Dr. Urberg's study has
led some experts to question niacin's primary role in lowering cholesterol. The study has even raised speculation that
niacin may actually enhance chromium's cholesterol-lowering
effects in the body, and not the other way around.

In San Diego, J.B. Gordon, M.D. used chromium in a form
called chromium picolinate together with niacin in ten patients. Each person took 200 mcg of chromium picolinate plus
one to two grams of niacin every day for four weeks. As a
result, blood LDL levels dropped by 27 percent, total choles-

terol levels dropped by 24 percent, and triglyceride levels dropped by 43 percent. These changes occurred without a reduction in the amount of HDL.[13]

We recommend that you take between 25 and 50 mg of a niacin-chromium supplement daily. Higher dosages should only be taken under a doctor's supervision. You should also consult your doctor if you have liver disease, peptic ulcers, diabetes, gout, or severe heart arrhythmia before taking *any* supplemental niacin.

The use of chromium-niacin supplements is definitely advisable for most older people who want to live longer without the complications of diabetes or heart disease. High levels of blood cholesterol have been linked to heart disease, the number-one killer in the United States today. The most effective and safest way to treat this common health problem includes exercise, a proper diet, and proper supplemention. In the next chapter, we'll look at bioflavonoids, vitaminlike substances that are essential to health, and in particular at a substance called OPC.

Chapter 9

The Power of
Vitamin C

M any people take vitamin C for protection against everything from colds to cancer. However, vitamin C doesn't work nearly as well by itself as when it is taken with other antioxidant substances. These substances include bioflavonoids and flavanols (OPC). They are not true vitamins in the strictest sense. Rather, they enhance the body's absorption of vitamin C, and should be taken with vitamin C.

Together, vitamin C and other antioxidents fight free radicals, the age-accelerating substances that we have discussed in Chapters 1 and 6. In this chapter, we will see how vitamin C and its helpers work together to protect the body from the effects of aging. We'll then see what makes a substance called OPC a particularly effective supplement.

VITAMIN C AND OTHER ANTIOXIDANTS:
A POWERFUL TEAM

Vitamin C (also known as ascorbic acid) came to the public's attention when Linus Pauling, a Nobel Prize-winning chemist, advocated its use in cold prevention. Vitamin C is an antioxidant, and therefore can help fight the free-radical damage that leads to such age-related disorders as heart disease and cancer. It bolsters the immune system and protects the body against the effects of stress. It is vital to tissue growth and repair, and to healthy gums. It also promotes the healing of wounds and burns.

The body cannot make vitamin C, which means it must be obtained from the diet. Good food sources include citrus fruits, berries, pineapples, tomatoes, cantaloupes, asparagus, broccoli, Brussels sprouts, radishes, kale, spinach, sweet peppers, and onions. The use of alcohol and tobacco will reduce vitamin C levels in the body, as can the taking of medications such as birth control pills, painkillers, steroids, antidepressants, and anticoagulants.

Bioflavonoids were first discovered in the white pithy part of citrus fruits. Since the human body cannot produce bioflavonoids on its own, supplies of these substances must come from the diet. Good food sources include grapes, rose hips, prunes, oranges, lemon juice, cherries, black currants, plums, parsley, grapefruits, cabbages, apricots, peppers, papaya, cantaloupes, tomatoes, broccoli, blackberries, peppers, and buckwheat.[1]

Bioflavonoids assist vitamin C in keeping collagen, the substance that cements the body's tissues together, in healthy condition. They are vital to the health of capillaries, the tiny blood vessels that connect arteries to veins. Bioflavonoids increase capillary strength and regulate how readily substances pass through the capillary walls. These effects can prevent bleeding and ruptures in the connective tissues, which builds a protective barrier against bacterial and fungal infections.[2-7]

Together, increased doses of vitamin C and bioflavonoids improve the symptoms of arthritis, rheumatism, and rheumatic fever. Diabetic retinopathy, a blood-vessel disorder of the eye that frequently affects diabetics who smoke, also responds to bioflavonoids.[8]

Bioflavonoids have been employed successfully to treat ulcer patients and those suffering from dizziness caused by an inner-ear disease called labyrinthitis. Weakness of the capillaries has been found to be a major factor in both of these ailments.[9] Bioflavonoid megadoses may also relieve asthma and protect the body against the harmful radiation effects of X-rays.[10] A wide range of other conditions, both major and minor, respond to bioflavonoids. These conditions include inflammations, diabetes, headache, viral infections, bee stings, atherosclerosis, high blood cholesterol levels, hemophilia, high blood pressure, stroke, varicose veins, hemorrhoids, pneumonia, skin ulcers, and pyorrhea (a gum inflammation).[11]

Scientists have found about 2,000 separate bioflavonoids. They include hesperetin, hesperidin, quercetin, catechin, and rutin. Research continues into the effects of these powerful substances.

OPC: THE MOST POWERFUL ANTIOXIDANT OF ALL

A substance related to the bioflavonoids, OPC, stands out as a most potent antioxidant. We will first explain what OPC is. We will then discuss how OPC, bioflavonoids, and vitamin C can be used together.

What Is OPC?

OPC (oligomeric proanthocyamidins) is found in all sorts of plant life. It is most highly concentrated in bark, stems, leaves, and skins, and thus is usually discarded before consumption, or is eliminated in cooking. Therefore, even people who eat a balanced diet are not likely to get enough OPC. Native Americans have used medicinal pine-bark teas for hundreds of years. We now know that these teas contain large amounts of vitamin C and OPC (see "Vitamin C and OPC Save Early Explorers" on page 90). Currently, the ability to isolate OPC from a plant source can only be assured through precise extraction processes.

Proanthocyanidins are contained in the plant pigments responsible for most scarlet, purple, mauve, and blue coloring in plants. Professor Jack Masquelier, Ph.D., the person who isolated OPC, discovered the importance of these substances while a student at the University of Bordeaux, France. He

Vitamin C and OPC
Save Early Explorers

During the winter of 1534–1535, explorer Jacques Cartier led a band of 110 weary Frenchmen through the forested wilds around the Saint Lawrence River in Canada. He and his men sought what they called the kingdom of Saguernay, where gold nuggets were said to be used as paving stones.

But the explorers, who were living off the provisions they had brought with them, found themselves growing progressively ill with various symptoms: weight loss, bone and joint aches, bleeding gums, loosening teeth, large bruises, utter fatigue. Twenty-five men died in their bedrolls, and were left in the deep snow—the others were too weak to even dig graves.

Then a Native American told Cartier that he and his men might be saved if they drank tea brewed with bark and needles from the Anneda tree. Cartier, who saw that the natives were in good health, did so. He and his men regained their health and eventually made their way home to France.

What Cartier and his men didn't know is that they were suffering from scurvy, a vitamin C deficiency. The tea relieved their symptoms because it was loaded with vitamin C and OPC.

found that proanthocyanidins are highly effective free radical neutralizers.[12] As we've seen, free radicals are responsible for a number of conditions, including cancer, cataracts, allergies, heart disease, peripheral vascular diseases, arthritis, diabetes, and various muscle and nerve problems.

The free radical-fighting effects of OPC can keep diseases associated with aging at bay. For example, hypoxia, an oxygen deficiency, in the brain tissues is likely to bring about a loss of mental function. OPC increases blood flow to the brain, which can in turn overcome hypoxia. It also keeps the blood from becoming sticky and clot-prone. These effects can delay the onset of hypoxia-induced mental difficulties.

Similarly, free radical damage associated with hypoxia can promote atherosclerosis and lead to clot formation. Together, these two processes can lead to heart attack. OPC may prevent hypoxia in atherosclerosis.

Tests indicate that the ability of the active substances in OPC to quench free radical activity is twenty times more powerful than that of vitamin C and fifty times more powerful than that of vitamin E.[13] These substances can increase the amount of vitamin C that enters the body's cells. They are also assimilated themselves into cell membranes. This allows them to serve as sentries, keeping various toxins out of the cells.

OPC also preserves vitamin C by blocking the formation of ascorbate oxidase, a chemical that destroys vitamin C. Vitamin C can actually become a damage-promoting pro-oxidant if exposed to certain minerals, such as iron or copper. OPC neutralizes these metals through a process called chelation (see Chapter 13) before they can degrade vitamin C.

A number of people have been helped by OPC and bioflavonoids. Wendy J., a nutritionist from Florida, has found that the use of these substances helped her avoid losing her sight. They reduced the bleeding and other forms of degeneration occurring in the retinas of her eyes. OPC has also eliminated her varicose veins, an effect noted in research studies.[14]

Richard N., a salesman from Illinois, found that both acne and severe sinus trouble have responded to OPC: "My sinuses are clear now. . . . Ordinarily at the change of the seasons, going from fall to winter, I get upper respiratory problems, but it has not happened . . . because of my taking OPC." Richard has also experienced a "general increase in well being." And William S., a food-store owner from Illinois, takes OPC to boost his immune system. He has found that it can remove toxins from the body, reduce swelling, and overcome circulatory problems.

Using Antioxidants and Vitamin C Together

OPC, bioflavonoids, and vitamin C should be taken together. As we've seen, they complement and enhance each other's effects. Vitamin C should be taken in divided doses of two to three grams (2,000 to 3,000 mg) a day. We recommend using the ester-C form. Avoid chewable vitamin C tablets, as they can cause tooth decay.

Vitamin C is nontoxic, even at high dosages, but amounts of 5,000 mg and up may produce loose stools and gas. You should not take more than 5,000 mg if you are pregnant. There is no truth to the common belief that high dosages of vitamin C cause kidney stones. However, you should see your doctor before taking vitamin C if you already have kidney stones, or if you have gout or chronic diarrhea. Also, under certain circumstances, your doctor may recommend intravenous vitamin C.

In dry form, OPC can be kept indefinitely at normal temperature. Due to OPC's superior water solubility, OPC is well absorbed and readily available to the body's tissues. It is generally well tolerated and nontoxic, even at elevated doses. There are no known medical conditions that would preclude the use of OPC.

OPC is sold in capsule or tablet form (see Appendix B). Generally, 100 to 200 mg a day is a good supplement dosage, although, as with most supplements, you should consult your doctor.

Bioflavonoids are sold in powder, liquid, capsule, and tablet forms. There are no known medical conditions that would preclude the use of bioflavonoids. Generally, 1,000 mg a day is a good supplement dosage, although up to 3,000 mg a day may be used in the treatment of an existing condition.

Vitamin C and other antioxidants are powerful weapons in the fight against free radicals. This makes them important parts of the antiaging arsenal. In the next chapter, we'll see how fiber, an old nutritional standby, is making a big comeback in the war on age.

Chapter 10

Enhancing Health
With Fiber

A n old idea is new again. Great-grandmother called it "roughage." Gastroenterologists call it "bulk." Most of us call it "fiber."

No matter what you call it, increased consumer demand for high-fiber foods has led manufacturers to consider many fiber sources for use in food production. That's because fiber in all forms can help keep the body healthy, and in ways that go beyond the simple relief of constipation. Even dietitians who are generally not in sympathy with the wholistic movement agree that fiber enhances health. It's the way to live a long life without any gastrointestinal difficulties.

Despite decades of emphasis on healthy foods, however, more than 60 percent of all American adults do not obtain enough dietary fiber. This lack of fiber causes digestive problems that affect more than a quarter of the population.

In this chapter, we will discuss the different types of fiber, and how fiber may prevent disease. We will then discuss the use of fiber as a normalizing agent.

A GLOSSARY OF FIBER FORMS

Fiber is actually an overall term for a number of different substances. We may better appreciate the function and benefits of food fiber by understanding some basic fiber terminology.

First, *dietary fiber* is the collective remains of the plant cells in food that resist digestion. Dietary fiber is the umbrella term for eight different substances: cellulose, lignins, hemicelluloses, waxes, pectins, mucilages, gums, and sterols. The first four components do not dissolve in water, and are collectively referred to as *insoluble dietary fiber.* The last four do dissolve, and are collectively called *soluble dietary fiber.*

Cellulose is the main structural fiber of the plant cell wall. *Lignins* are resin-like materials that make the cell wall more rigid. *Hemicelluloses* are complex substances that tie cellulose fibers together. *Pectins, mucilages,* and *gums* are carbohydrates found in some plants. *Waxes* and *sterols* are some of the miscellaneous components found in dietary fiber.

When scientists speak of *crude fiber,* they mean the residue of a food sample analyzed according to a particular method of chemical digestion. Unfortunately, only some of the cellulose and a little of the lignins and hemicelluloses are measured by this procedure. Food composition tables often give the crude fiber content because this analysis is the most traditional and widely used method of determining the amount of fiber in foods. However, crude fiber analysis does not accurately reflect the true amount of indigestible material in food products. It probably represents only about one-third of the dietary fiber present in foods.

FIBER AND DISEASE PREVENTION

The connection between fiber and health was made through the observations of a British scientific team working in Uganda. The work of this team, led by Denis Burkitt, M.D., prompted researchers to take a closer look at the correlation between a low-fiber diet and the many degenerative diseases experienced by people in modern societies, including diverticulitis, hemorrhoids, varicose veins, appendicitis, bowel cancer, and irritable bowel syndrome.

Dr. Burkitt spent many years studying the diseases, living habits, and diets of rural Africans. He observed that there was a low incidence of the degenerative diseases that plague modern societies. As a surgeon, he noticed during operations that Africans generally had a lot less body fat than Britons.

Dr. Burkitt also noted that African foods and elimination habits differed greatly from those prevalent in the United States and Europe. The stools of Africans were larger and softer, which made them easier to eliminate. These stools were also passed with considerably more speed. In Africa, Dr. Burkitt noted a transit time from ingestion to elimination of nine hours.[1] On the other hand, a study was done by a U.S. Food and Drug Administration advisory review panel on bowel health in the United States. The panel found that 95 percent of all Americans experience satisfactory elimination just once every seventy-two hours. Among the elderly, it sometimes takes more than two weeks for food to pass from one end of the system to the other.

In Great Britain, Dr. Burkitt observed that stools were generally small, hard, and difficult to expel, and that they sometimes damaged the intestinal lining. He also became aware that many of the people who were hospitalized were suffering from diseases, such as diverticulitis and bowel cancer, that were almost unknown in a traditional society such as rural Uganda.

What made the difference? Dr. Burkitt decided that diet was the reason. In modern societies, fiber is refined out of carbohydrate food. The consumption of refined foods is partially responsible for the relatively high rate (40 percent) of obesity in modern societies. It is also responsible for the prevalence of constipation. In traditional societies, people consume two and a half times more fiber than people in modern societies by eating starchy staples such as brown rice, potatoes, maize, and casaba. People in traditional societies also eat very little meat.

Older people are also at risk for constipation if they do not drink enough fluid (at least eight to ten glasses of water a day). Low fluid intake can lead to the formation of dry, hard stools that are difficult to pass. This type of constipation may actually trigger diarrhea, which occurs when the bowel wall releases large amounts of fluid as the result of prolonged irritation.

Small, hard stools and slow elimination times mean that toxic waste products build up in the bowel. Eventually, this waste buildup lowers the individual's immunity to disease. Various microbes, such as *Giardia lamblia*, can take hold (see Chapter 11). The toxic buildup damages the large intestine's sensitive lining, leading to such problems as colitis and even bowel cancer. Straining to eliminate hard stools can also damage the intestinal lining. This can lead to hemorrhoids and diverticulitis, in which the bowel wall develops inflamed bulges.

Fiber normalizes or regulates bowel function, aiding in the formation of soft, smooth, easy-to-eliminate stools. Soluble fiber absorbs the excess water that produces loose stools. This reduces constipation and the toxic buildup that accompanies it. (For a full discussion of natural laxatives and internal cleansing, see Chapter 11.)

For example, Neil Painter, M.D., a senior surgeon at Manor House Hospital in London, used dietary fiber to successfully treat patients with advanced diverticulitis. Dr. Painter put 70 patients on a high-fiber diet. At the start of the study, the patients reported 171 symptoms. At the end, bowel habits had improved significantly, and the symptoms were reduced by more than 88 percent.[2]

If all fiber did was eliminate constipation and its harmful effects, it would be well worth adding fiber to your diet. However, fiber also promotes health in other ways. To see how the two different kinds of fiber affect the body, see Table 10.1.

The poor diet and sedentary lifestyle in modern societies often lead to an excess of cholesterol in the bloodstream. Normally, cholesterol is used in many important ways throughout the body. Under certain conditions, however, this excess cholesterol can form fatty deposits called plaques on the inside of the arteries. This process, called atherosclerosis, can lead to a heart attack or stroke.

Table 10.1. Overall Effects of Fiber

Effect	Soluble Fiber	Insoluble Fiber
Reduces blood cholesterol/ fats	Strong effect	Weak effect
Satisfies appetite	Strong effect	Strong effect
Stabilizes blood sugar	Strong effect	No effect
Reduces bacterial toxins	Strong effect	Strong effect
Speeds bile acid excretion	Strong effect	Weak effect
Speeds elimination	Weak effect	Strong effect
Absorbs toxins	Weak effect	Strong effect
Softens stools	Weak effect	Strong effect
Improves bowel disorders	Weak effect	Strong effect

One of the ways the body uses cholesterol is in the creation of bile acids. Such acids are made in the liver and released into the intestines to help the body digest fat. Soluble fiber soaks up bile acids and removes them from the body, which forces the body to pull more cholesterol out of the bloodstream for bile acid production. Thus, the use of fiber can help lower the amount of cholesterol, especially the "bad" LDL cholesterol, in the blood. Fiber also promotes the creation of the "good" HDL cholesterol that helps prevent the development of plaques. (For a fuller discussion of LDL and HDL cholesterol, see Chapter 9.)

Fiber's effect on bile acid creation also helps to prevent the development of gallstones. Bile is stored in the gallbladder, a small sac underneath the liver. Increased bile production leads to a freer flow of bile through the gallbladder. As a result, stones are less likely to develop.

According to James Anderson, M.D. of Lexington, Kentucky, daily consumption of the dietary fiber contained in a bowl of oatmeal and three bran muffins will lower blood pressure by 10 percent.[3] That is because eating more fiber tends to reduce obesity. The less body fat you have, the less work your heart has to do in pumping blood through your blood vessels. As a result, blood pressure drops.

Fiber has also been shown to help diabetics, whose bodies cannot adequately control levels of glucose, or blood sugar. Fiber slows the absorption of glucose from the small intestine, which reduces the diabetic's dependence on insulin, the body's glucose-control chemical.

USING FIBER FOR OVERALL HEALTH

Both insoluble and soluble natural fibers absorb many times their weight in water in the intestinal tract. For example, wheat bran, which is predominately insoluble fiber, absorbs three times its weight in water. Psyllium, which is predominately soluble fiber, absorbs 40 times its weight in water. This water absorption softens and increases the bulk of the stool, which in turn increases pressure against the intestinal muscles, facilitating and regulating transit through the intestines.

When soluble fibers are mixed with water, they become soft and bulky. Taken in sufficient quantity (20 to 40 grams) throughout the day, the mixture fills the intestines with a moist, soft mass that clings to the intestinal walls and removes old material that may have accumulated. That allows the body to eliminate waste buildup.

A number of foods contain healthy amounts of fiber. The prune, with 1.7 grams of fiber for every ten prunes, is a well-known fiber food. A large variety of other raw and dried fruits are high in fiber, including apples, pears, bananas, blueberries, dates, grapes, papayas, mangos, pineapples, and raspberries. To see which foods contain the greatest amounts of specific types of fiber, see Table 10.2.

For information on the use of fiber in constipation relief, see Chapter 11. However, if you want to make fiber a regular part of your overall health plan, it is a good idea to eat whole-grain breads and bran cereals, and to cut down on your intake of refined flours and sugars. It also wouldn't hurt to add one to two tablespoons of unprocessed bran to your

Table 10.2. Food Sources of Fiber

Fiber	Source
Insoluble Fiber	
Cellulose	Course bran, unpeeled apples and pears, canned peas, fresh carrots
Hemicellulose	Bran cereals, whole-grain breads, beets, eggplant, radishes
Lignin	Pears, toasted whole-grain breads, potatoes
Soluble Fiber	
Pectin	Bananas, oranges, apples, potatoes, cabbage, carrots, grapes
Gums, mucilages	Oatmeal, sesame seeds, psyllium seeds, beans, psyllium-containing bulking agents

daily diet. You can sprinkle it on cereals, stews, and casseroles, or mix it into a full glass of water.

To avoid gas and loose stools, do not add too much fiber to your diet all at once. Add fiber gradually to give your intestines a chance to adapt to it. You should increase your fluid intake, since fiber is most effective when sufficient moisture is present. See your doctor before increasing your bran intake if you have ulcerative colitis or regional ileitis.

Dietary fiber has long been used in the treatment of constipation. It increases stool weight because of its water-holding properties. Transit time, the time taken for passage of food material from ingestion to elimination, is greatly reduced on a high-fiber diet. A faster transit time helps prevent bowel problems such as diverticulitis, colitis, and hemorrhoids. We now know that fiber can be used in treatment plans for other conditions, such as high cholesterol levels, gallstones, and diabetes. These are all conditions that tend to occur more frequently as a person ages. So fiber can help keep your intestines—and the rest of you—healthy.

In the next chapter, we will take a closer look at constipation, a common problem of advancing age, and at the intestinal cleansers that can fight constipation.

Chapter 11

Natural Laxatives and Internal Cleansers for Bowel Health

I n Chapter 10, we saw how the modern-society diet of highly refined, low-fiber foods has led to an epidemic of chronic constipation. As a result, Americans spend more than half a billion dollars a year on laxatives. We also saw how chronic constipation can lead to many of the diseases associated with aging, such as colon cancer and diverticulitis. This happens because toxic materials build up in the intestines when food does not move through them fast enough. That is why wholistic practitioners say, "Death begins in the colon."

The accumulation of intestinal toxins can adversely affect your health by poisoning your body's cells, disrupting its chemical reactions, and displacing necessary nutrients. This causes your body's chemistry to go out of balance, which in turn causes the loss of your natural defense mechanisms. Reduced resistance to the absorption of toxins, in turn, results in further toxin accumulation.

Thus, constipation relief is an important part of any anti-aging program. In this chapter, we will first look at the importance of bowel health. We will then discuss the reasons for constipation, and examine the different internal cleaners that may be used to correct this common problem.

THE INTESTINAL TRACT AS AN ECOSYSTEM

The intestinal tract is an enormously complex and dynamic ecosystem that contains millions of tiny plants and animals, many of which are necessary for proper digestion. They are collectively referred to as the gut flora. In a normal tract, there is a healthy balance among the gut flora, the food that enters the tract, and the secretions produced by the tract. At any given moment, the character of the intestinal tract reflects variations in any of these three components.

The intestinal tract, like the rest of the body, is protected by the immune system, which has two important but conflicting jobs. It must allow the body to absorb needed substances, such as nutrients, but it must also keep out harmful substances, such as bacteria. That means the gut flora has to be kept in healthy balance. How can you help your body do this? By assisting your body to rid itself of substances produced by harmful gut flora. This allows the body to avoid the toxins that cause chronic intestinal inflammations. Chronic irritation of the intestinal walls can make the body sensitive to certain foods and chemicals, and can lead to ill health.

The key to bowel health is to keep food moving through the intestinal tract. Food that moves along quickly cannot stagnate and create toxic substances. Remember, the bowel is a muscular tube. Muscles in the bowel, as with all muscles of the body, work more efficiently when given sufficient work to do. Thus, if your bowel is largely full, the muscles will propel this bulk through at a proper rate of speed. The movement of food through the intestinal tract can be compared to the movement of toothpaste through a tube. It takes little pressure to squeeze toothpaste out of a new tube. But when the tube is largely empty, it takes a great deal of pressure to squeeze out the remaining contents.

Ideally, it should take twelve to fifteen hours for food to move from one end of the intestinal tract to the other. Unfortunately, many people do not pass food through their systems quickly enough. The modern diet consists of many highly refined, almost totally absorbed foods (see Chapter 10). This leaves inadequate bulk in the intestinal tract.

CONSTIPATION AND ITS CAUSES

When waste material moves too slowly through the large intestine, and thus is passed infrequently, a condition of constipation exists. (For more information on bowel transit time, see Chapter 10. For a general anticonstipation program, see "A Twenty-Point Program for Constipation Relief" on page 104.)

There are three principal types of constipation: atonic, spastic, and dyschezic. *Atonic constipation,* or inactive colon, is common among the elderly and the infirm. It also occurs in younger persons who have developed faulty habits because of the absence of convenient toilet facilities or preoccupation with other matters. Sometimes several days may pass without a bowel movement or a feeling of the desire to defecate. This can result in loss of appetite, bad breath, and mental sluggishness.

Atonic constipation is best corrected by a balanced diet rich in fresh vegetables and fruits. Sufficient fluid intake is needed to prevent the development of hard, dry stools. Some grains have laxative properties because of their indigestible bulk. Finely ground brans from oats, wheat, rice, and some other cereals are effective bulk laxatives. Psyllium seed is a safe and effective bran substitute. Since a B-complex vitamin deficiency contributes to constipation, a supplement providing 50 mg of the full complement of B vitamins ought to be taken for nutritional support.

As a rule, laxatives should be avoided for atonic constipation because some of them may irritate the colon and aggravate the constipation. Mineral oil was once taken extensively as a laxative, but it is messy and absorbs vitamin A out of the intestines.

Spastic constipation is often referred to as irritable colon and shows up in nervous persons living under high tension. Their bowel movements are variable and irregular, but periods of

A Twenty-Point Program for Constipation Relief

Three European physicians have developed a twenty-point program to aid those suffering from constipation. Dr. Horst Jungmann, Dr. Berthold Thomas, and Dr. Hans Schoberth have devised a program of point values for particular bowel-stimulating activities. Every day, you should select a combination of activities with point values that equal twenty when totaled:

- Eat only brown bread such as whole wheat, never white—6 points

- Establish regular bowel habits, same time and place—6 points

- In the evening, eat a tablespoonful of bran in yogurt—5 points

- Attempt a bowel movement as soon as you feel the need—5 points

- Eat at least three servings of vegetables—4 points

- Kneel, exhale completely, draw in the stomach, and force it out as powerfully as possible; repeat three times—4 points

- Drink white wine rather than red to avoid the tannins—3 points

- Drink at least four glasses of water—3 points

- Eat breakfast earlier to have time to enjoy the meal—3 points

- Chew every mouthful twice as long as you usually do before swallowing—3 points

- Lie on your back, draw up the knees, hold, and then stretch legs straight; repeat ten times—3 points

- Bend forward before an open window; repeat five times—3 points

- Swim using the breaststroke as much as possible—3 points

- Drink room-temperature beverages to avoid slowed digestion—2 points

- Include muesli and fresh fruit in the diet—2 points

- Keep to the same bowel routine on weekends and holidays—2 points

- Lie flat on your stomach, raise your torso, and then lower it again (all with the mouth open); repeat ten times—2 points

- Contract and expand the buttocks rhythmically for six seconds—2 points

- While on your back, relax the abdomen and drum it with the fingers—2 points

- Do breathing exercises directly after rising in the morning—2 points

constipation predominate. Hemorrhoids are a frequent complication. Rest, mental quiet, and any of the vast numbers of mild sedative herbs may be useful. The sedative herbs lower the activity level of the bowel and other organs. Therefore, they tend to have a calming, moderating, or tranquilizing effect. Sedative herbs include blue cohosh, camomile, belladonna, evening primrose, foxglove, pusatilla, and many more. Like any other drug, some herbal sedatives have side effects. For example, belladonna can produce blurring of vision and difficulty in passing urine. See an herbalist for advice on using sedative herbs.

Dyschezia is the term for difficult defecation, a form of constipation caused by the retention of stool. The production of dry, hard stools can result from eating mostly junk foods, such as French fries, pretzels, candy, and white-flour breads. These stools are irksome to pass, and sometimes passage doesn't occur for a week. The solution lies in an improved diet of uncooked vegetables, whole-grain cereals, and fresh fruits with a high water content, such as melon. Colon-cleansing laxatives can also help.

Not the least of the problems involving constipation is the possibility of parasite infestation. Every fourth person in the United States has one or more parasites living somewhere in his or her body, mostly within the intestinal tract. These parasites generally come from unclean water or raw food meat. Symptoms include bloating, gas, indigestion, fatigue, abdominal cramps, and alternating diarrhea and constipation.

Some parasites cause irritation and interfere with bodily functions. Others destroy tissue and release toxins. Human parasites include:

- *Giardia lamblia*, a protozoa, the most common parasite. It can cause gastrointestinal disturbances, food intolerance, chronic fatigue syndrome, and immune system dysfunction. Giardiasis should always be treated, even in individuals without symptoms, because of the risk of activation and spread to other parts of the body, and to other people.

- *Entamoeba histolytica*, an amoeba. It causes bowel disturbances, food intolerance, chronic fatigue, and immune system dysfunction. The extent of illness caused depends upon the strain of amoeba present. If a heavy infestation with an especially invasive strain occurs, entamoeba can migrate to the liver and brain.

- *Cryptosporidium*, a parasite with worldwide distribution. Patients with strong immune systems can experience a self-limiting diarrhea. There may be abdominal discomfort, loss of appetite, fever, nausea, and weight loss. In people with suppressed immune systems, acutely severe diarrhea and generalized symptoms are typical. Death could even occur from dehydration. The organism can spread to other parts of the body.

- *Blastocystis hominis,* a parasite that generally produces mild intestinal upset and diarrhea. It can be problematic for people with poor immune system function.

- *Endolimax nana,* a common protozoa that generally is harmless. However, it can cause arthritis in individuals with active inflammatory disorders.

The presence of parasites can be determined by a laboratory test done on the stool. (For information, see Appendix B.) There is an urgent need for internal cleansing when parasites are present.

TYPES OF INTERNAL CLEANSERS

Some foods can have a cleansing effect on the bowel. Acidophilus milk contains *Lactobacillus acidophilus,* a healthy gut flora species. When mixed in a 1 to 9 ratio with buttermilk, acidophilus may have a laxative effect. Chlorophyll, the green coloring of plants, also aids in maintaining bowel health when taken as spirulina, wheat grass, chlorella, green barley essence, or another purified form. These green foods act as deodorants, antiseptics, and tissue builders. Green foods are best when used in liquid form as a drink or in soup.

The person who wants to normalize bowel movements or remove parasites can use a variety of internal cleansers. There are several different types of internal cleaners:

- Bulk-forming laxatives

- Stimulant laxatives

- Stool-softener laxatives

- Lubricant laxatives

- Enemas

- Internal-cleansing exercises

The U.S. Food and Drug Administration (FDA) has approved all of the cleansers discussed in the following sections, except where noted. All dosages listed below are for adults *only*. See the package of each individual product for children's dosages.

Bulk-Forming Laxatives

Internal cleansers of the bulk-forming type increase the colon's bulk volume and the water content of stools. Water softens stools and makes them easier to pass. The FDA views them as among the safest types of internal cleansers. (Also see Chapter 10 for information on fiber.)

Bulk-forming laxatives should be accompanied by from two to four quarts of liquids (water, juice, herbal teas, soup, skim milk, and cereal beverages substituting for coffee and regular tea) each day. The beverage provides the active bulk-forming ingredient with sufficient liquid to soften and expand the stools. The liquid also guards against the rare possibility that the laxative might become impacted in the digestive tract. These laxatives include the following:

- Dietary bran, especially when consumed in foods such as oat-bran bread, whole-wheat bread, and other whole-grain breads, and in breakfast cereals containing from 2.7 to 6.5 grams of bran flakes per 100 grams of cereal. The FDA says that 6 to 14 grams of bran—¼ ounce to ½ ounce— each day is an effective laxative. Bran tablets are not nearly as effective, since they may not be completely broken down before being eliminated.

- The cellulose derivatives methylcellulose and carboxymethylcellulose sodium are safe and effective when 4 to 6 grams a day are taken. One must drink a minimum of eight ounces of water each time a cellulose derivative is taken.

- Karaya (sterculia gum), a vegetable gum, is safe and effective in a 5- to 10-gram daily dose. Drink water immediately after taking karaya in order to avoid the risk of bowel obstruction.

- Malt soup extract is a powder prepared from partially ger-minated barley grains. It contains 73 percent maltose, 7 percent protein, and 1.5 percent potassium, plus lesser amounts of various minerals. Malt soup acidifies the in-testinal tract, which helps to relieve constipation. The safe and effective dosage is 12 to 64 grams daily with water.

- Polycarbophil can bind and absorb sixty times its weight within the colon. The safe and effective dose is 5 grams daily. Drink a full glass of water with each dose.

- Psyllium preparations—psyllium and blond psyllium seeds, psyllium seed husks, psyllium hydrophilic mucilloid, psyl-lium hemicellulose, plantago seed, plantago ovata husks—bind and hold water. Psyllium preparations are taken with water in dosages ranging from 2.5 to 30 grams per day.

- Bentonite is a ground-up volcanic ash found deep in the earth. It swells up to twelve times its original volume when added to water. As a colon cleanser, its action is physical, not chemical. Because of its absorptive qualities, bentonite can remove bacteria, parasites, environmental pollutants, and other contaminants from the intestinal tract. However, it can also remove friendly bacteria, so these useful organisms should be replaced after the constipation is resolved. Additionally, bentonite takes nutrients out of the bowel and they also have to be replenished. The FDA has made no ruling on bentonite.

Stimulant Laxatives

Stimulant laxatives act directly on the walls of the large in-testine, the small intestine, or both intestines. These sub-stances activate peristalsis, the wavelike muscle contractions of the intestines, to move the stool along. Some stimulant lax-atives irritate the intestinal wall, while others stimulate the nerves to start peristalsis.

According to the FDA, these laxatives must be used with caution. The FDA warns that stimulant laxatives should not be employed often, and not daily for more than a week. Overdosage or persistent use can produce side effects, which include dependence on the laxatives for proper bowel movement. Body fluids and essential body salts (electrolytes) may also be depleted. Stimulant laxatives can also produce severe spasmodic bowel pain and increased mucus secretion, and, in some people, cause loose stools.

The common herbal stimulant laxatives are the anthraquinones—aloe, cascara sagrada preparations, and senna preparations. They act mainly in the large intestine. Another anthraquinone, danthron, is synthetic. They all may discolor urine, turning acid urine yellowish-brown and alkaline urine reddish-violet. The senna products are more potent than cascara, according to the FDA, and may bring on greater abdominal discomfort. Cascara sagrada, an herb with a long history of use for chronic constipation, aids the secretion of bile and increases peristalsis. If taken with bentonite or psyllium, it moves these bulk formers through the colon, as well. See Table 11.1 for recommended dosages.

Castor oil, that old standby, more than meets the modern standards of a stimulant laxative. One dose of 15 to 60 ml will completely clear out the lower bowel. Castor oil's laxative effect comes from ricinoleic acid, a substance that is not produced until the oil reaches the small intestine.

There are other stimulant laxatives. Dehydrocholic acid comes from cholic acid, a natural bile acid. It increases the water content of bile. It is safe and effective at doses of from 750 to 900 mg per day. Prune concentrate dehydrate has been only conditionally approved as a laxative by the FDA, although prunes are widely accepted as a home remedy for constipation. Chinese rhubarb contains chemicals that are related to active laxative ingredients found in aloe, cascara sagrada, and senna. The FDA has given Chinese rhubarb only conditional approval.

Elderberry/elderflower drink is a highly effective bowel stimulating laxative that has diuretic properties. A full program of elderberry internal cleansing includes both elderberry drink and tablets, along with herbal teas, a bulk-forming

Table 11.1. Daily Dosages for
Various Anthraquinone Products

Product	Daily Dosage
Aloe	120 mg to 250 mg
Cascara sagrada preparations	
Fluid extract	2 ml to 6 ml
Casanthranol	30 mg to 90 mg
Bark	300 mg to 1,000 mg (1 gram)
Tablets	1 to 3
Senna preparations (single dose)	
Fluid extract	2 ml
Senna fruit extract	3.4 grams to 4 grams
Senna leaf powder	500 mg to 2,000 mg (2 grams)
Senna pod concentrate	600 mg to 1,000 mg (1 gram)
Senna syrup	8 ml
Sennosides A and B crystalline	12 mg to 36 mg
Danthron	75 mg to 150 mg

colon cleanser, and other products in a complete body detox-ification program (see Appendix B). Elderberry internal cleansing can also stimulate weight loss. A book on the sub-ject is also available (see *The Healing Powers of Elderberry Internal Cleansing* in Appendix A).

Stool-Softener Laxatives

The most commonly used drug in this class is Colace (do-cusate sodium), which is available in capsule, syrup, or liq-uid form. It is a relatively safe drug that softens hard stools, making them easier to pass. It is prescribed for patients with certain conditions, such as anal or rectal problems, to avoid pain on defecation. Possible side effects include throat irritation, nausea, a bitter taste in the mouth, and, on occasion, rash. However, the use of Colace rarely results in side effects. Pregnant or nursing women should consult their doctors before taking Colace.

Lubricant Laxatives

Lubricant laxatives make the intestinal tract and stool more slippery, which permits easier passage of stool. The time-honored intestinal lubricant is mineral oil, which may be taken orally or inserted into the rectum. It has been discovered, however, that organically grown, unrefined, cold-pressed food oils are more effective as internal cleansers than mineral oil, and do not produce its side effect of removing fat-soluble vitamins, such as vitamin A, from the colon.

Food-quality oils include flaxseed (linseed), almond, virgin olive, pumpkin seed, sesame, toasted sesame, sunflower, safflower, canola, walnut, and peanut. These oils smooth the intestinal tract, soften the stool, and lubricate the colon mucosa. They are nonirritating, and are not only safe but also supply vast amounts of nutrients.

Enemas

Enemas employ liquid introduced through the rectum to remove stool and promote healing. There are three types of enemas that accomplish internal cleansing: the nystatin retention enema, the garlic evacuant enema, and the coffee evacuant enema.

Nystatin is a prescription drug that kills the disease-causing yeast *Candida albicans* in order to eliminate this common source of yeast infection. (See *The Yeast Syndrome* in Appendix A.)

The garlic and coffee evacuant enemas both help remove stool from the lower colon. The garlic evacuant enema requires two capsules of deodorized aged garlic extract that have been opened and emptied into two quarts of warm water. The coffee evacuant enema uses four rounded tablespoons of regular-grind coffee that has been boiled or perked in two quarts of water. The coffee should be the color of weak tea.

Take either the coffee enema or garlic enema, or interchange the two on alternate days. To give yourself an enema:

1. Lie on your left side and let in one-half to one cup of solution.

2. Massage the lower left side of your abdomen. Work hard on any lumps or ridged areas that you feel.

3. After four or five minutes of massaging, let in more water. Continue to massage across the abdomen and down your right side.

4. Do not retain the liquid if you feel the need to eliminate, but try to hold the solution for approximately fifteen minutes. Simply start over if your retention interval is too short.

5. Expel waste matter and observe if brown-, grey-, or black-flecked mucus is present. Look for parasites.

Enemas should not be overused. If the constipation is not relieved after several days, see your doctor.

Internal-Cleansing Exercises

One of the easiest ways to cleanse the bowel is to jump on a mini-trampoline called a rebounder (see Appendix B). This exercise places no trauma on the joints, offers deep cleansing of the cells, and provides a general physiological lift. Bouncing on the rebounder effectively helps to move food along the intestinal tract. It can also stimulate the lymphatic system, which rids the body of toxins such as dead and cancerous cells, nitrogenous wastes, fat, infectious viruses, heavy metals, and other assorted wastes. (For more information on rebound exercises, see *Jumping for Health* in Appendix A.)

Slantboard exercises will help stimulate bowel movement. Every day, lie on your back on the slantboard. Then stretch your abdomen by putting your arms above your head and then lowering them to your sides. Repeat fifteen times.

Another bowel-stimulating exercise is done before you get out of bed. Lie on your side and thrust your abdominal muscles in and out several times. Then turn onto your back and draw up your knees. Using your fingertips, massage your abdomen with slow, circular motions from the right groin up to just under the ribs and across to just above the navel before moving down the left side. Repeat several times. Finally, toss off the covers and stretch out your legs. Raise the right leg *very* slowly as high as you can, and then lower it. As you're lowering your right leg, raise your left leg, keeping both legs about an inch off the mattress. Gradually increase the repetitions to six.

As we've seen, maintaining a clean colon can keep toxins from building up in the body and leading to many of the diseases often associated with aging. A clean colon can also help the body absorb the maximum amount of nutrients, and one of the most nutrient-dense foods available is yogurt. In the next chapter, we'll see how this simple food can help promote longevity.

Chapter 12

The Longevity Potential of Yogurt

When he was eight years old, it was Emanuel Ramone's job to make yogurt for his family. He would boil milk in a big clay pot, and cool the pot slightly by placing it in a closed kitchen cabinet with some cold water. Once it was tepid, he would add a little yogurt culture saved from the previous day's batch, and stir a few times. Finally, he would pour the milk into smaller containers, wrap each container in a blanket, and place the containers in an oven with the heat off. In a couple of hours, yogurt would form.

Emanuel Ramone has continued to follow this procedure. He eats a pint of his yogurt daily—plain, with no sweeteners such as fruit, sugar, or honey. The only difference is that today, Emanuel Ramone is well into his 100s.[1] And while homemade yogurt isn't the only reason for his longevity, it doesn't hurt.

In this chapter, we'll first see what yogurt is. We'll then discuss why yogurt is good for you, and how you can ensure that your yogurt contains plenty of the active ingredient—a colony of bacteria.

WHAT IS YOGURT?

Around the planet, fermented milk is a staple food in many
cultures. Milk ferments when certain kinds of bacteria prolif-
erate in it, causing the milk to thicken and curdle so that
the taste turns sour. By far, the *Lactobacillus* family of bacteria is the largest family of milk-fermenting organisms. These
friendly bacteria turn the milk into compounds that both alter
the milk's chemistry and produce health benefits for the person who consumes the final product. The specific strain of
bacteria used determines what specific type of fermented milk
will be produced (see Table 12.1).

Table 12.1. Fermented Milk Products

Milk Product	Bacteria Type
Acidophilus milk	*Lactobacillus acidophilus*
Bulgarian milk	*L. bulgaricus*
Cheeses	*L. brevis, L. bulgaricus, L. casei, L. helvetics, L. lactis*
Kefir	*L. caucasicus*
Koumiss	*L. bulgaricus*
Yakult	*L. casei*
Australian yogurt*	*L. bulgaricus, S. thermophilus, L. acidophilus*

*Australian yogurt has all three types of bacteria. Other types of yo-
gurt have one or two of these strains.

Of all the products in Table 12.1, yogurt may be the oldest health food. It was mentioned in the Book of Genesis,
and was eaten by both the ancient Egyptians and the ancient
Hebrews.[2]

Yogurt can be made from regular milk, skim milk, sweet
cream, buttermilk, sour cream (both cultured and acidified),
whey, and cottage cheese (both cultured and acidified). While
usually made from soured cow's milk, yogurt is also derived

from the milk of sheep, pigs, goats, and other domestic animals.

When yogurt is produced commercially, the initial milk or milk product may be homogenized. It must be pasteurized or ultrapasteurized prior to the addition of the *starter*, which contains the fermenting bacteria. Flavoring ingredients may be added after pasteurization. To extend the shelf life of the food, manufacturers sometimes heat-treat the yogurt after culturing is completed. However, this destroys not only spoilage organisms, but also the *Lactobacillus* organisms that give yogurt its healthful properties.

Since the yogurt starter is the most important ingredient, it is carefully monitored. A starter is evaluated using a number of performance factors, including rapid acid development; typical yogurt flavor, body, and texture; and survivability of the culture during storage.[3] Strict criteria, established by the National Yogurt Association, are used to ensure that yogurt that has not been heat-treated contains the proper amount of active cultures.[4] There are three categories of recognized yogurt product: yogurt, low-fat yogurt, and nonfat yogurt.

WHY YOGURT IS GOOD FOR YOU

Nobel laureate Elias Metchnikoff was one of the first scientists to explore the longevity benefits of yogurt. In his 1908 book, *The Prolongation of Life*, he wrote: "From time immemorial human beings have absorbed quantities of lactic microbes by consuming in their uncooked condition substances such as soured milk, kefir, sauerkraut, or salted cucumbers which have undergone lactic fermentation. By these means they have unknowingly lessened the evil consequences of intestinal putrefaction."[5]

Subsequently, Dr. Metchnikoff developed a lactic acid-producing microbe that he named *Bulgarian bacillus* (*Lactobacillus bulgaricus*) that, when fed to mice, caused the animals to thrive. Compared with mice fed a normal diet, the *Lactobacillus*-fed mice lived longer, gave birth to more offspring, and exhibited the least intestinal putrefaction. Each day, the scientist himself drank a pint of the special "sour milk" he had invented.

Part of yogurt's health benefit is that it is extremely digestible. The bacteria in yogurt break down milk proteins during the fermentation process, which allows yogurt's nutrients to be readily available. This makes yogurt a high-quality source of animal-derived protein. That is especially important to the estimated two-thirds of the Earth's population that is *lactose intolerant*. Lactose is the sugar present in milk, a sugar that lactose-intolerant people cannot digest because they lack the digestive enzyme lactase. This results in cramps, bloating, or diarrhea when milk is consumed. However, lactose-intolerant people can eat yogurt because almost no lactase is required to digest it.

Yogurt also provides a healthy dose of calcium, a mineral that is not only essential for strong bones and teeth, but that also performs other important functions in the body (see Chapter 5). Each eight-ounce serving of yogurt delivers 37.5 percent of the 1,000 mg of calcium you should get each day. (Cup for cup, yogurt offers one third more calcium than milk.) The bacteria in yogurt also produce the B vitamins niacin, pyridoxin, cobalamin, and folic acid. And because commercial yogurt is often thickened with extra milk solids, it generally contains more protein than milk does.

However, yogurt's most important health benefit lies in the bacteria themselves. These friendly bacteria suppress toxin production by a family of unfriendly bacteria called *Enterococci*. The toxin produced by these bacteria can cause inflammation of the mucous membranes within both the small and large intestines. Yogurt can thus protect the intestines against infection, such as the infection that results in travelers' diarrhea.[6] One *Lactobacillus* strain, *L. acidophilus*, is able to suppress the growth of *Escherichia coli* and *Salmonella typhimurium*, two foodborne disease organisms.[7]

Yogurt's friendly bacteria protect against illness by overwhelming the disease-producing organisms that are always present in the intestines. This includes organisms such as *Candida albicans*, which promotes yeast infections, and *Staphylo-*

cocci, which produce boils and other infections. Such harmful organisms can multiply rapidly under unfavorable conditions, especially if the body's own friendly intestinal organisms, called gut flora, have been weakened.

For example, physicians will often recommend acidophilus yogurt to patients who are prescribed antibiotics. Antibiotics disrupt the balance between friendly bacteria and harmful invaders by killing off the helpful microbes and allowing noxious, drug-resistant microbes to prevail. Diarrhea can be the uncomfortable result, but *L. acidophilus* in yogurt may prevent the condition by recolonizing the intestines with friendly organisms. Another type of friendly bacteria that offsets the overall killing effects of antibiotics is *Bifidobacteria*, which is also found in some types of yogurt.

Vaginal yeast infections are often accompanied by a decline in levels of the *L. acidophilus* that is normally found in the vagina. This can occur as the result of conditions, such as diabetes, that upset the vagina's natural balance. Since there is evidence that acidophilus fights the growth of *C. albicans*, which is responsible for most vaginal yeast infections, most wholistic physicians recommend that patients use acidophilus to clear up the condition.

One study at the Long Island Jewish Medical Center in New York found that women with vaginal yeast infections who consumed eight ounces of acidophilus-containing yogurt every day for six months had fewer recurrences than women with infections who ate no yogurt.[8] Researchers in Israel found that applying up to three teaspoons of acidophilus-containing yogurt directly into the vagina every day produced an immediate and lasting improvement in twenty-eight of thirty-two pregnant women who had bacterial vaginal infections.[9]

Yogurt also has cancer-preventing properties. Part of this effect lies in yogurt's ability to fight harmful bacteria, since these bacteria can promote the development of carcinogens, or cancer-causing substances, within the intestines. Yogurt helps prevent the conversion of precarcinogens to carcinogens. It also protects the intestines from the harmful effects of ni-

trosamines, chemicals that are found in some types of pre-
served foods.

Yogurt's anticancer effects have been proven in studies.
When yogurt is injected into the implanted cancers of mice,
tumor growth is suppressed in the short term, although the
survival rate is not significantly increased in the long term.
Yogurt has also been shown to boost several immune-system
components in mice. Milk shows no such effect.[10,11] European
studies have found that people who eat large amounts of yogurt or other fermented milk products do show a lower incidence of breast cancer.[12] Researchers from the New England
Medical Center in Boston fed twenty-one patients milk containing *L. acidophilus* every day for four weeks. As a result,
the cancer-promoting bacteria in their stools were three times
less active than when the same people were given milk that
did not contain *L. acidophilus*.[13]

Some strains of *L. acidophilus* have shown an ability to soak
up cholesterol in the intestines. This helps reduce the amount
of cholesterol that circulates in the bloodstream, which is important because a high cholesterol level can be a factor in
heart disease. Unfortunately, other strains aren't nearly as effective, and there is no way to tell if the strain (or strains)
in the yogurt you buy is predisposed to absorbing excess
cholesterol.[14]

MAKE SURE YOUR YOGURT IS ACTIVE

As we've seen, yogurt is good for you—but only if it contains active *Lactobacillus* cultures. If the manufacturer has heat-
ed the yogurt to hold down its tartness and extend its shelf
life, the microbes won't be lively, or will be killed altogether.

Some strains are stronger than others. The most robust mi-
croorganism is *L. acidophilus*. It endures passage through the
stomach better than two of the more frequently used yogurt
cultures, *L. bulgaricus* and *S. thermophilus*. *L. acidophilus* is not
used as often because it is more acidic and tangy, and thus
less suited to the American market, where consumers prefer
a sweeter yogurt.

The best way to insure that you have the healthiest yogurt is to make it yourself, using one of a variety of yogurt makers on the market. The starter is the most crucial component in making high quality yogurt. You can usually acquire the starter from a health food store or a manufacturer who specializes in culturing the appropriate organisms. Once you buy the initial starter, you can keep your own starter from batch to batch. The instructions that come with the yogurt maker will tell you how.

Your other option is to buy your yogurt. If you are watching your weight, get a low-fat or nonfat brand. But watch out for the sugar content. Flavored yogurts can contain as much as nine teaspoons of sugar per cup, and your body will readily turn sugar into fat if you eat more sugar than you burn off in exercise. Your best bet is to buy unsweetened yogurt and then add fruit and just a teaspoon or two of sugar or honey.

One reason that so many commercial yogurts are so sweet is that yogurt is normally eaten as a breakfast food or as a snack. But yogurt is a versatile food. It can be a healthful substitute for sour cream in dips, dressings, and other cold dishes. You can also use yogurt in sauces, casseroles, and baked goods. Remember, though, that once you heat yogurt, the bacteria are either killed or weakened. So while yogurt may be a healthier ingredient than sour cream in a casserole, for instance, you will still need to eat uncooked yogurt in some form to get its full health benefits.

You also have to be concerned with the number and strain of lively organisms in the yogurt you eat. It's the only way to be certain that the yogurt is doing you any good. Consequently, you should ask the distributor or, better yet, the manufacturer what organisms are in the brand you buy, whether the yogurt has been heat-treated (which can kill the bacteria), and how many bacteria there are in each serving. Sometimes, you can find this information on the container.

There are many reasons to eat yogurt. It can provide you with a healthy dose of nutrients, protect your intestines from infection, and bolster your immune system against cancer. Some strains can even absorb excess cholesterol. But yogurt must contain active cultures to be effective. Carefully check the yogurt you buy, or make it yourself. In the next chapter, we will see how a treatment called chelation therapy can help protect your health and prolong your life.

Chapter 13

Using Chelation Therapy to Promote Longevity and Treat Alzheimer's Disease

Two of the most debilitating conditions associated with aging are heart disease and Alzheimer's disease. However, there is a safe and effective treatment that can prevent or reverse much of the damage done by these conditions. It is called *chelation therapy.*

Chelation (pronounced "key-lay-shun") therapy has been known to American organized medicine for years, yet only about a thousand physicians have taken advantage of its enormous potential. It has been the subject of a large government-approved study (see Appendix A). This amazingly simple treatment can help reduce the incidence of degenerative diseases, the types of diseases that kill 90 percent of those who die each year in industrialized countries.

Chelation therapy is the treatment of choice whenever disease arises from an interruption of blood flow or from heavy metal poisoning. In this chapter, we will first see how chelation therapy works. We will then look at how it can be used to treat cardiovascular disease and Alzheimer's disease, and how you can use one version of chelation therapy at home to help prevent these conditions from developing in the first place.

HOW CHELATION THERAPY WORKS

In Chapter 4, we learned how certain toxins called heavy
metals are common in our polluted environment, and how
the build-up of heavy metals within the body can impair normal functioning. Chelation therapy works by pulling toxic
heavy metals and other harmful substances from the tissues,
which restores normal cell function.

What exactly is chelation? Chelation is the ability of some
substances to form a molecular "claw" that can bind onto
other substances. Together, the two substances form a *chelate*,
which has different chemical properties than those of either
substance. In this manner, the chelating agent can latch onto
noxious substances such as heavy metals and draw them out
of the body.[1]

There are two forms of chelation therapy: intravenous and
oral. *Intravenous chelation*, in which the chelating agent is introduced into the patient's vein via a needle, must be done
under a doctor's supervision. Each session lasts from three
to four hours, and the patient is carefully monitored. Many
sessions may be required, depending on the patient's condition at the time treatment is started. This is necessary because chelation is a slow process, for two reasons. First, many
toxic substances within the body tend to be very tightly
bound to protein. Second, substances such as heavy metals
can cause a variety of symptoms if they are removed from
the body too quickly (see Chapter 4).

The other option, *oral chelation*, can be used by healthy people who wish to prevent disease. However, we must emphasize that if you are ill with a serious disease, such as
heart disease, or if you have symptoms, such as angina, that
are associated with serious disease, oral chelation therapy will
not help you very much. *Oral chelation therapy is no substitute
for intravenous chelation therapy.* Although chelating orally certainly does work to reverse hardening of the arteries, it works
more slowly and less effectively than intravenous therapy. (To
find a physician who administers intravenous chelation therapy, see Appendix B.) Sometimes, oral chelation is used be-

fore intravenous treatments are started. This allows the patient's body to accept a greater volume of intravenous fluid.

We must also emphasize that chelation therapy is *not* a substitute for a healthy lifestyle. Chelation, whether intravenous or oral, must be used along with a proper diet, appropriate exercise, and stress reduction. Otherwise, its effects will be minimal.

A number of substances have chelating properties. Intravenous therapy uses several substances, including ethylene diamine tetraacetic acid (EDTA); ethyl-glycol-bis-beta-amine-ethyl-ether-N, N-tetraacetic acid (EGTA); and dimethyl sulfoxide (DMSO).[2] Oral chelation therapy uses a variety of foods and nutritional supplements, some of which are described starting on page 128.

CHELATION THERAPY AND CARDIOVASCULAR HEALTH

As we saw in Chapter 5, calcium is a mineral that is vital to health. However, under some conditions, the body can build up excess calcium. This is called *hypercalcemia*, and it can occur as the result of parathyroid or thyroid disease, or certain types of cancer. It can also occur if excessive amounts of vitamin D or milk and antacids are ingested. This excess calcium is a factor in arterial hardening, since it serves as a cementing agent within deposits of cholesterol called plaques that are found on the walls of diseased arteries. EDTA can bind to this excess calcium and take it out of the body.

One of chelation therapy's most obvious benefits is in the treatment of coronary artery disease, in which plaques form in the arteries that supply blood to the heart itself. By helping to reverse the formation of plaque in these arteries, chelation therapy reduces the risk of heart attack. For the same reason, chelation therapy can help prevent strokes, which are often caused by clots becoming stuck within hardened arteries in the brain. Chelation therapy can also help patients with other conditions that involve diseased blood vessels, such as phlebitis and varicose veins.

Chelation therapy can produce remarkable results. Charles R., 64, of Illinois was taking a number of cardiovascular medicines, including vasodilators, blood pressure pills, and diuretics. He had constant thirst and fatigue, a feeling of heaviness in his chest, and pain in his legs upon exertion. The leg pain, called intermittent claudication, is caused by insufficient blood flow to the legs.

After only five intravenous chelation treatments, Charles's intermittent claudication disappeared. After twenty infusions, he was able to throw away his heart and blood pressure medicines. Friends remarked that he looked a dozen years younger, too. Thereafter, Charles went on a program of oral chelation.

Henry B., 49, of Missouri had a history of increasingly severe chest pain. It so disabled him that he could no longer walk across the street. Even worse, the heart medications he was taking had rendered him impotent.

Immediately after starting chelation therapy, Henry found he needed a marked decrease in medications. His angina disappeared completely, and he was no longer impotent. He could rake leaves, take long walks, and resume his normal business activities without any physical problems. Henry's doctor weaned him off cardiac drugs and replaced them with oral chelation agents.

CHELATION THERAPY AND
ALZHEIMER'S DISEASE

Doctors have established a link between toxic metal accumulation in the brain and Alzheimer's disease, a form of dementia that causes progressive memory loss, confusion, and restlessness. In 1980, two doctors at Mount Sinai Medical Center in New York discovered that not only did aluminum appear in the brains of Alzheimer's disease victims, but that it was present in precisely those tangled brain cells that characterize the disease.

One of those doctors, Daniel Perl, M.D., head of Mount Sinai's Department of Neuropathology, investigated diseases associated with aluminum poisoning and found a baffling wave of degenerative brain disease on the Pacific island of Guam. About 10 percent of Guam's local population dies of degenerative brain diseases. There are high levels of aluminum in the drinking water there, and Dr. Perl repeatedly found the metal in the brains of the deceased.[3,4]

Aluminum toxicity is an increasing problem in the United States. Aluminum enters our food supply from aluminum cans and cookware, and the use of aluminum foil in wrapping acidic foods such as tomatoes. It is found in processed cheese, pickles, baking soda, and cake mixes, and in common medicine-cabinet items such as buffered aspirin, douches, antacids, and antiperspirants.[5]

Aluminum is known to be a potent cross-linking agent, which means that it can damage brain function. It also causes free radical damage within the nerve cells. As we said in Chapter 1, free radical damage can accelerate aging in all of the body's tissues, including the brain. In a series of brilliant studies, Donald R. McLachlan, M.D., at the University of Toronto, and his coworkers, showed that aluminum can cause a dementia similar to Alzheimer's in laboratory animals, and that aluminum will travel to the brain no matter where it enters the body.[6] Research suggests that the body may absorb more aluminum when a chronic calcium deficiency is present.[7] (For more information on calcium, see Chapter 5. For more information on toxic metal poisoning, see *Toxic Metal Syndrome* in Appendix A.)

By using chelation therapy for victims of Alzheimer's disease, cardiologist H. Richard Casdorph, M.D., Ph.D., of Long Beach, California, has reversed the symptoms of dementia. In a study of fifteen patients, the treatment was successful in reducing memory losses and in increasing intelligence. In a journal article, Dr. Casdorph said, "Intravenous infusions of disodium EDTA are shown to be an effective form of therapy for various states associated with abnormal [brain] blood flow. This is particularly noteworthy in view of the fact that medical science has no other effective treatment for most of these conditions [Alzheimer's]."[8]

ORAL CHELATION: THE AT-HOME THERAPY

As we've said before, if you have a serious illness, we strongly recommend that you consider taking intravenous chelation therapy under a doctor's care. However, there are certain foods, vitamins, and other substances that, when taken orally, can remove toxins from the body. Supplementation with these substances is called oral chelation.

Oral chelation can help retard the development of degenerative diseases such as atherosclerosis and cancer. It can also slow the aging process overall. Oral chelation agents work by reversing, stopping, or preventing destructive chemical reactions within cells. This causes the cells to release toxic wastes, and thus keep the body in a healthy state of balance. Oral chelation can also help reduce the fatty deposits that form on the walls of the blood vessels, although its action is not as strong or thorough as that of intravenous chelation.

Oral chelation is also a good followup to intravenous chelation, especially when used in conjunction with healthy changes in lifestyle. Vladimir M., 63, a diplomat from Romania, suddenly started experiencing sporadic chest pains while visiting relatives in New York. He didn't think they were symptoms of heart disease because he had always eaten a healthy diet. However, he had taken almost no routine exercise for twenty years, and was quite badly overweight.

The chest pains became frequent enough that Vladimir was forced to seek medical attention. He was given therapy for angina pectoris, uncontrolled high blood pressure, and general circulatory problems. He also received intravenous chelation treatments and help in losing weight.

By the end of the intravenous infusion series, Vladimir showed such remarkable progress in his health that he was put on a monthly maintenance program of oral chelation nutrients and antioxidants. He continued on this program after returning home.

There are at least 100 nutritional supplements that act as oral chelation agents. Some of them, such as vitamin C, are in common use. Others are not so common. Some of these oral chelators are described here. For more information, see *The Chelation Way* in Appendix A.

Some oral chelators are vitamins. *Vitamin E* is a fat-soluble vitamin that occurs in high concentrations in cold-pressed vegetable oils. It is an antioxidant that can fight the damage caused by free radicals (see Chapters 1 and 6) and retard cellular aging. It improves the health of the red blood cells, which carry oxygen throughout the body. This increases stamina and endurance. Vitamin E also dilates the blood vessels to increase blood flow, inhibits clot formation and strengthens the tiny blood vessels known as capillaries. Elsewhere in the body, vitamin E promotes production of linoleic acid, an essential fatty acid, and helps improve eyesight. It also prevents the oxidation of both the pituitary and adrenal hormones.

Vitamin C is a water-soluble vitamin that has antioxidant properties. It promotes the activity of folic acid, a B vitamin. It protects the B vitamins thiamine, riboflavin, and pantothenic acid, and vitamins A and E, against oxidation. Vitamin C stimulates calcium metabolism and promotes the actions of the amino acids phenylalanine and tyrosine.

Vitamin C works best when taken with *bioflavonoids*, water-soluble substances that are sometimes referred to as vitamin P (see Chapter 9). They are established oral chelators that tend to prevent bleeding, ruptures, and disruptions of the capillaries.

The *ascorbates* are chemical salt derivatives of vitamin C, which is also called ascorbic acid. The ascorbates promote the activity of other oral chelators, such as zinc. They react in the bloodstream with magnesium, zinc, calcium, and other minerals. The vitamin C acts as a chelating agent for the particular mineral and forms magnesium ascorbate, zinc ascorbate, etc., giving rise to a natural human chelation mechanism.

Some minerals also act as chelators. The *aspartates* are substances that are chemically related to minerals such as magnesium and potassium. For example, the magnesium in magnesium aspartate helps to displace the calcium that binds the material within fatty deposits on blood-vessel walls. Magnesium aspartate and potassium aspartate taken together may increase the heart's pumping action. *Magnesium* itself is important for the health of the heart muscle and coronary blood vessels. (For more information on magnesium, see Chapter 5.)

Zinc is a building block of twenty-five enzymes, chemicals that promote chemical reactions within the body. It is also essential for cellular reproduction, and for the normal functioning of the male reproductive system. (For more information on zinc, see Chapter 6.)

Manganese is a trace mineral that stimulates the body's use of various vitamins. It is also needed for the production of fatty acids.

Some herbs can act as chelation agents. *Aged garlic extract* is a new form of an herb that has been used medicinally for thousands of years. Garlic can help lower high blood pressure as well as elevated levels of cholesterol and fat in the blood. Garlic exhibits a binding action with lead, mercury, cadmium, and other heavy metals. This property makes it an excellent chelating agent. The aged extract is available in tablet, capsule, and liquid forms that have been processed to reduce the garlic odor.

Some fatty acids also have chelating properties. *Eicosapentaenoic acid* (EPA) is a fish oil that protects the body against heart disease and strokes. It is an omega-3 fatty acid, a class of essential fatty acids that is required for production of substances that control blood clotting and arterial spasms. EPA improves blood viscosity, lowers blood cholesterol levels, and reduces blood fat levels. It can also improve functioning of the nervous and immune systems.

Evening primrose is an herb that yields the fatty acids linoleic acid and gamma-linoleic acid. Oil of evening primrose helps the body to manufacture substances that are essential for cell structure growth.

There are a variety of other oral chelation agents that do not fall into any of the standard categories. *N,N-dimethylglycine* (DMG) helps promote chemical reactions within the body. It is manufactured by the body and is also found in some foods, including cereals, beets, seeds, and organ meats. Supplementing with DMG increases cellular efficiency, and combats both fatigue and a lack of oxygen in the tissues. It is useful in cases of alcoholism, diabetes, sexual dysfunction, and atherosclerosis.

Protomorphogens help promote protein synthesis and cell repair, especially when the body is under stress. Protomorphogens are found in glandular tissues, and are present in supplemental glandular extracts. These extracts are available in tablet, capsule, droplet, or powdered form.

Spirulina is a species of algae. This small plankton provides complete vegetable protein that contains large amounts of vitamins, minerals, digestive enzymes, trace elements, cell salts, and chlorophyll.

Glutathione is an amino acid, or protein building block. It is a free radical scavenger.

Health is a state of wholeness based on the body's ability to maintain an equilibrium between internal and external forces. Healing is the body's innate ability to restore bodily equilibrium and wholeness. Chelation therapy promotes healing by encouraging the body to regain its natural state of balance. In the next chapter, we look at the healing capacities of herbs.

Chapter 14

Restoring Vigor With Herbal Remedies

Many people find they lose vigor as they age. Indeed, fatigue is one of the most common complaints in doctors' offices. Sometimes, fatigue and listlessness are associated with an underlying medical condition, such as diabetes or depression. Sometimes, they are associated with disrupted sleep patterns, especially since sleep problems are more common among older people. Or they may occur for no identifiable reason. In any case, fatigue and a general lack of vigor can drain the pleasure and enjoyment out of life.

While there are numerous medications that have a stimulating effect, stimulant herbal remedies may provide a safe, natural lift. Most of them can also help improve specific conditions. In this chapter, we'll first examine the ideas behind herbal medicine, and than take a look at some herbs with stimulant properties. (For a list of tonic herbs, see "Herbal Tonics" on page 136.)

THE REBIRTH OF HERBAL MEDICINE

Whether they grow on land (such as ginseng) or in the sea (such as kelp), all herbs are plants. To the extent that we consume vegetables, fruits, spices, and other vegetation, we are taking in herbs as nutritional sources. However, it has been long recognized that some plants have a greater effect on the body than others. These plants are regarded as herbal medicines.

For thousands of years, herbal medicine was the only medicine. Over 80 percent of the world's rural population still relies on herbalists for medical treatment today. Herbs not only enhance the workings of our bodies, but they also help normalize metabolic processes that have gone awry. They allow the body to heal itself.

When conventional Western medicine was first developed, doctors stopped using herbal remedies in favor of stronger, chemically produced drugs. It was thought that this would put medicine on a more scientific footing. However, the scientific community now knows more about the chemical properties of herbal supplements than it did in the past. It also realizes that strong medicines can have strong side effects. Thus, doctors have learned to accept herbal medicines for their real contributions to nutrition and health. No longer do people consider herbal stimulants and other types of botanicals as magical in their actions. Instead, we know that by aiding the body nutritionally and biochemically, herbs can reverse many ailments.

In China, herbal medicine never fell into disuse. Chinese herbal healing began with the acknowledged father of ancient herbal medicine, Shen Nung, who developed a system of healing about 3490 B.C. Shen Nung's system involves five elements in the human body—metal, wood, fire, water, and earth. Each element stands for some basic natural process; for example, fire represents activity. These elements have to be kept in balance in order to avoid illness. The various medicines used in this system are ascribed specific characteristics and prescribed according to the characteristics of the patient's illness. For instance, if the patient has an inflammation or an infection (that is, a local "fire"), then an herb having a "water" characteristic is prescribed to counter the hot spot.

Chinese medicine is also guided by the belief that the

physical world is only a visible form of the universal cosmic energy known as the Tao. The idea is that the human body must be aligned to the Tao to be in complete health. Certain herbs, such as ginseng (page 137), are seen as being able to adjust the body so that it is more completely aligned with the Tao.

The earliest written record of the *Shen Nung Pen Tsao*—Shen Nung's works as handed down verbally over centuries—is the book of *Pen Ching*, written by Tao Hung-Ching (A.D. 456–536). It contains descriptions of 365 herbs. It was only the first in a long line of Chinese books devoted to medicine. Today, the Chinese are learning to incorporate the best of Western medical technology, such as the latest surgical techniques, into their system of ancient knowledge.

No matter where they come from, stimulant herbs can help counteract fatigue and improve overall vigor. Most are useful in treating specific problems. They are valuable for older people because they can help enliven processes that may start to slow down with age.

In general, herbal remedies are gentler and safer than their chemical cousins. However, any substance that is strong enough to help is also strong enough to harm if used incorrectly. Always follow the label instructions. Do *not* exceed the recommended dosage. If you have any negative reactions, or any reactions that take you by surprise, stop taking the herb and speak with your doctor. While the herbs in this chapter are available to the general public, we strongly recommend that you use them under a doctor's supervision, especially if you have a pre-existing condition such as heart disease. If your doctor is unfamiliar with herbal medicine, we suggest that you consult a wholistic or naturopathic physician, or an herbalist.

CHINESE HERBAL REMEDIES

The herbs discussed in this section are available through a Chinese herbalist or a Chinese herb shop (see Appendix B). The exception is ginseng, which is widely available. A vari-

Herbal Tonics

The herbs discussed in this chapter tend to have fairly pronounced effects. But some herbal agents give increased
vigor, energy, and strength by stimulating nutrition, and thus
act in a more subtle manner. These herbs, called *tonics*,
can be found in health food stores. You can learn more
about them from herbal manuals, or by talking to an herbalist. They include:

- European Centaury (*Erythraea centaurium*)
- False Unicorn Root (*Chamaelirium luteum*)
- Gentian (*Gentiana lutea*)
- Myrrh (*Commiphora myrrha*)
- White Poplar (*Populus tremuloides*)

ety of ginseng is used in traditional American herbal medicine, but is discussed under this heading for ease of reference.

Asiatic Cornelia Cherry

A member of the magnolia family, Asiatic cornelia cherry
(*Schizandra chinensis*) is listed in the *Pen Ching* as a high-grade
herb with a pungent, bitter, and overall salty taste. It has an
astringent action on the lungs and a nourishing effect on the
kidneys. It encourages the secretion of fluids, controls excessive sweating, and terminates diarrhea. In traditional Chinese
medicine, Asiatic cornelia cherry is used to treat difficult
breathing, to stop coughing, to end thirst and dryness of the
mouth, to relieve insomnia, to eliminate amnesia, and to end
excessive perspiration. It has antimicrobial and liver protective effects. The toxicity of Asiatic cornelia cherry is low to
nonexistent.

Ganoderma Mushroom

Ganoderma mushroom (*Ganoderma lucidum*) is a fungus that grows on coniferous and deciduous trees. It is employed in traditional Chinese medicine. Ganoderma can increase the sex drive and reinforce the body's resistance to infection by acting as a detoxifying agent. It has a low order of toxicity.

Ginseng

One of the most well-known of all stimulant herbs is ginseng. There are several different varieties of ginseng, but three are most often used medicinally: Asian ginseng (*Panax ginseng*), American ginseng (*Panax quinquefolium*), and san-ch'i ginseng (*Panax pseudoginseng var.notoginseng*). Siberian ginseng (*Eleutherococcus senticosus*), a thorny shrub that grows in Siberia, China, and Korea, has properties similar to those of ginseng. The ginsengs have been used in China and elsewhere in the Orient as stimulants for more than 4,000 years. References to them date back to 2600 B.C. and appear in *Pen Ching*. In ancient times, ginseng was reserved for the emperor and the imperial household.

As verified in modern laboratories, for centuries the Chinese have considered *Panax ginseng* the ultimate adaptogen. An adaptogen is a drug that doesn't cause many side effects; is able to increase one's resistance to adverse influences through a wide range of physical, chemical, and biochemical factors; and usually brings about a normalizing action in the body and mind irrespective of the nature of the problem.[1] American ginseng is also an adaptogen. The various ginsengs are mild in their effects, causing neither drug dependency nor tolerance following extended periods of usage.

Ginseng, when taken with gotu kola (page 140) and cayenne (page 139), can act as a potent restorative and decelerator of the aging process. This combination herbal formula also is useful for regulating the blood pressure and blood sugar levels, supporting the pituitary and adrenal glands, increasing energy, prolonging endurance, and increasing a sluggish libido. Ginseng promotes health in both men and women, since it aids in regulating the endocrine, or hormone-producing, systems of both sexes. If you suffer from diabetes or hypoglycemia, high blood pressure, or heart disease, see your doctor before taking ginseng. (For more information, see *The Ginseng Book* in Appendix A.)

Traditionally, Siberian ginseng is taken by Chinese herbal exponents for restoration of vigor, return of memory, improvement of sexual performance, increase of appetite, and prolongation of longevity. Over a thousand published clinical journal articles attest to Siberian ginseng's usefulness in increasing productivity, enhancing physical strength and endurance, improving visual acuity and hearing, and increasing resistance to infections. It is one of the least toxic herbal agents known.[2] San-ch'i ginseng is a weak tonic. It is generally used to disperse unwanted blood, such as in bruises.[3]

Lovage

In traditional Chinese medicine, lovage (*Ligusticum linneaus*) is thought to promote the flow of *Qi*, or vital energy, and is used to build one's life force. It invigorates blood circulation, dispels wind, and controls pain. Chinese doctors use lovage to relieve headache, abdominal discomfort, joint pain due to cold, and spasms of the tendons. They also prescribe it for amenorrhea (absence of menstrual flow) and for other menstrual disorders. Do not take excessive dosages of lovage, as this can cause kidney problems. People with pre-existing kidney conditions should *not* take this herb at all.

Privet

In Chinese medical practice, privet (*Ligustrum lucidum*), a member of the olive family, is given to treat fever, deafness, dizziness, palpitations, insomnia, and constipation. It lessens both neurosis and depression. Extracts of the plant are found to stimulate white blood cell formation in patients with low white cell counts due to chemotherapy or radiation treatment. The bark and leaves are the medicinal parts; the berries are poisonous.

Wolfberry

Wolfberry is a name given to about one hundred plant species growing chiefly in temperate and warmer regions. Its stimulative properties make the herb particularly useful for offsetting radiation sickness, such as that caused by radiation treatment or other such exposure. It strengthens the liver and kidneys. Wolfberry also promotes sperm production and blood formation. The *Lycium* wolfberry species, in particular, is employed by Chinese herbal doctors in relieving vertigo, coughs due to tuberculosis, and diabetes.

OTHER STIMULANT HERBS

The herbs in this section are available either through a health care provider or through health food stores. There is an American version of the Chinese herb ginseng. Still, for ease of reference, all forms of ginseng are dealt with on page 137.

Black Pepper

Black pepper (*Piper nigrum*) has a stimulative, tonic, antiperspirant, and fever-reducing effect. This is an active stimulant, especially to the gastrointestinal tract, for which it may be taken as a substitute for cayenne. It can be used to treat colic, fevers, flatulence, indigestion, rheumatism, sore throat, and gum trouble.

Cayenne

Cayenne (*Capsicum minimum*) works as a tonic and stimulant on the immune and circulatory systems, and on other body systems. Cayenne regulates the blood flow from the head to the feet so that it becomes more uniform. Its effects on the heart muscle occur immediately, then gradually extend to the arteries, capillaries, and nerves. While the frequency of the pulse is not increased, it does become more powerful. Cayenne may be used as a gargle for sore throat, tonsillitis, and halitosis, and is beneficial for arthritis and rheumatism.

Cayenne contains a number of important nutrients, including calcium, manganese, potassium, and the B-complex of vitamins, especially B_2 and B_6. All of these nutrient components enhance the herb's overall stimulative qualities.

Cloves

Cloves (*Caryophyllus aromaticus*) are taken for their antiseptic, antispasmodic, and antinausea effects. This herb increases blood circulation, promotes digestion and nutrition, raises the body temperature, and tightens the skin. It stimulates the excretory organs to disinfect the kidneys, skin, liver, and bronchial mucous membranes. It is the most powerful of the aromatic and carminative herbs. Oil of cloves works wonderfully for treating toothache and as a liniment, and a drop or two can cover the taste of bitter or sour herbal drinks. However, pure clove oil can be an irritant. Dilute it with olive oil before external use. Essential oil should not be taken internally except under a doctor's supervision. Also, use cloves sparingly until you are certain that you are not allergic to them.

Ginger

Ginger (*Zingiber officinale*) is a stimulant that may be used as a substitute for cayenne when the latter, a more effective herb, is unavailable. Since it excites the bowels, ginger acts as a mild laxative. It helps cleanse the colon (see Chapter 11), stimulate the circulation, and reduce spasms and cramps arising in the gut. It is also an excellent antinausea remedy. However, it can cause stomach distress if taken in excessively large quantities. (For more information, see *The Ginger Book* in Appendix A.)

Gotu Kola

Gotu kola (*Hydrocotyl asiatica*) is known as the memory herb, because it tends to stimulate general brain function and creative thinking in particular. When taken regularly, gotu kola increases one's learning ability. It has been employed as a treatment for nervous breakdown and senile dementia not caused by Alzheimer's disease. Gotu kola tends to reduce mental fatigue and forgetfulness. It can also eliminate depression, elevate sex drive, and decrease fatigue. This mildly bitter herb contains several nutrients, including magnesium and vitamin K. However, it may induce skin irritation if applied externally.

Horseradish

Horseradish (*Cochleria armoracia*) is one of the most active stimulant herbs, especially for the digestive organs, kidneys, skin, and circulation. It gives a feeling of pleasant warmth in the stomach and stimulates intestinal action. It also increases the flow of urine. Horseradish is taken to relieve a number of conditions, such as bronchitis, constipation, cough, hoarseness, indigestion, jaundice, malnutrition, neuralgia, low blood pressure, sinus trouble, sluggish liver and stomach, and vomiting. Do not ingest too much horseradish at one time.

Peppermint

Peppermint (*Mentha piperita*) is one of the great stimulative herbs and is a marvelous antispasmodic. Peppermint strengthens the nerves and heart muscle, assists in digestion, cleanses and tones the entire body, and soothes the stomach. Peppermint may very well be the most extensively used medicinal herb in the world. One caution is that peppermint may interfere with the absorption of iron from food and supplements.

Prickly Ash

Prickly ash (*Zanthoxylum americanum*) bark has general and cardiac stimulant qualities. It is a tonic and antiseptic, and can calm the nerves. The action of this stimulant is slower than cayenne, but its effects are more permanent. It can remove obstructions from every part of the body. It can increase circulation and produce warmth during chills. It is effective in cases of asthma, cold extremities, colds, colic, diarrhea, edema (water retention), problems with the female reproductive system, flatulence, liver problems, backache, throat inflammations, sores in the mouth, toothache, ulcers, and wounds.

There's no reason to let a lack of energy keep you from enjoying an active life. If you are always feeling tired and washed out, visit your doctor to find out whether or not you have some underlying medical condition. If you don't, then you may want to try one of the herbs we have discussed in this chapter. Just be sure to ask your doctor or herbalist for advice and follow the label instructions. In the next chapter, we will see how hydrogen peroxide, an old first-aid standby, is being handled in a new way.

Chapter 15

Fighting Disease
With Intravenous
Hydrogen Peroxide

Hydrogen peroxide—a substance found in raindrops, most medicine cabinets, and the human body—has physicians around the world excited about its ability to cure both degenerative and infectious diseases. This includes diseases that become more common as individuals age, such as heart disease, emphysema, and arthritis.

Today, hydrogen peroxide is being employed by physicians in an altogether different way—by intravenous infusion in exceedingly small amounts. Doctors who administer intravenous hydrogen peroxide, Dr. Kurk among them, are reporting excellent results.

In this chapter, we will first see how hydrogen peroxide works within the body. We will then see how doctors are using intravenous hydrogen peroxide (also referred to as *biooxidative therapy*) to help patients with a number of difficult-to-treat medical conditions. It is important to note that this is *not* an over-the-counter therapy; please read "Do Not Drink Hydrogen Peroxide" on page 144.

HOW HYDROGEN PEROXIDE
WORKS WITHIN THE BODY

In Chapters 1 and 6, we have discussed how free radicals can damage the body's cells. Free radicals are a product of

Do Not Drink
Hydrogen Peroxide

Every day, thousands of people drink glasses of diluted, food-grade hydrogen peroxide. Why? They believe that oral hydrogen peroxide will put oxygen into the bloodstream, and that this extra oxygen will eliminate arthritic pain and assist the body's immune system. Some individuals have promoted this practice as a treatment for various degenerative diseases.

Unfortunately, the body does not process hydrogen peroxide taken orally in the same way as hydrogen peroxide taken intravenously. The fatty materials often present in the stomach, particularly when they are in the presence of iron salts and ascorbate, will reduce hydrogen peroxide to chemicals[1,2] that can harm the linings of the stomach and intestines. Serious consequences include ulcers, an overgrowth of intestinal cells called duodenal hyperplasia, and both benign and malignant tumors. These effects occurred in laboratory mice fed hydrogen peroxide over a ten-week period in concentrations as small as 0.8 percent.[3]

To avoid the risk of developing these serious conditions, *do not drink hydrogen peroxide*, whether it is labeled "food-grade" or not. Internal hydrogen peroxide must always be administered by a doctor.

---

1. Rowley D.A. and Halliwell B. Formation of hydroxyl radicals from hydrogen peroxide and iron salts by superoxide and ascorbate-dependent mechanisms: relevance to the pathology of rheumatoid disease. *Clinical Science* 64:649–653, 1983.

2. Bielski B.H.J., Arudi R.L., and Sutherland M.W. A study of the reactivity of HO_2/O_2—with unsaturated fatty acids. *Journal of Biological Chemistry* 258:4759–4761, 1981.

3. Ito A., Watanabe H., Naito M., and others. Induction of duodenal tumors in mice by oral administration of hydrogen peroxide. *Gann* 72:174–175, 1981.

one type of oxidation, which is a general name given to chemical processes that involve oxygen. Rust formation and fire are two other examples of oxidation.

But oxidation has its positive side, too, and is a necessary reaction within the body's cells. If oxygen reactions do not occur within the body for more than a few seconds, death ensues. The brain thrives on oxygen. The body uses oxidation as its first line of defense against bacteria, viruses, yeasts, parasites, and other unfriendly microorganisms.

A number of substances cause oxidation in the body, but the most important of these is hydrogen peroxide. Hydrogen peroxide is an unstable compound that is readily broken down into water and oxygen. This process makes water and oxygen available to the body's cells.

You can see this process take place whenever you put the hydrogen peroxide in your medicine cabinet on a wound. The foam that forms consists of oxygen bubbles, and it is the oxygen that disinfects the wound. A small amount of hydrogen peroxide can supply large amounts of oxygen to the tissues.

Hydrogen peroxide has various functions within the body. It is an integral part of the system that helps the body to regulate all cell membranes. It functions as a regulator of hormones such as estrogen, progesterone, and thyroid hormone. It is necessary for the regulation of blood sugar and the production of energy in all cells. It helps control nearly all chemical reactions related to the brain and nervous systems. Finally, it is a vital part of the immune system. Quite clearly, hydrogen peroxide is a substance the body cannot live without. Medical scientists are discovering that the role hydrogen peroxide plays within the body is far more complex than previously realized.

The number of important functions carried out by hydrogen peroxide explains why bio-oxidative therapy works; it simply supplies more of a substance the body uses anyway. Hydrogen peroxide is a powerful oxidizer that affects toxic materials invading the body. For example, just one set of clinical effects that doctors have observed after intravenous hydrogen peroxide therapy would best be described as "oxida-

tive detoxification." The oxidative benefit includes the elimination over time of fatty material from the blood vessel
walls.[1] Repeated treatments have been found by investigators
to remove the plaques that cause atherosclerosis in blood vessels, and to increase the elasticity of arteries and veins.[2,3]

USING HYDROGEN PEROXIDE
TO FIGHT DISEASE

Intravenous hydrogen peroxide is not a new therapy. Rather,
it has been proven medically safe and beneficial since the beginning of this century.[4,5] As far back as 1920, patients with
influenza pneumonia were treated with hydrogen peroxide infusions with very good results.[6] This therapy has been studied at many major medical research centers throughout the
world, with as many as fifty scientific articles on the subject
being published each month.

Charles H. Farr, M.D., Ph.D., of Oklahoma City, Oklahoma,
became a strong supporter of bio-oxidative therapy after he
discovered that patients with chronic obstructive lung disease
or asthmatic bronchitis respond remarkably well to carefully
administered intravenous hydrogen peroxide. Dr. Farr, who is
considered to be the father of intravenous hydrogen peroxide, spearheaded the formation of a nonprofit physicians' educational and research organization called The International
Bio-Oxidative Medicine (IBOM) Foundation. (For more information about the group, including information about doctors
in your area who use this treatment, see Appendix B.)

Intravenous hydrogen peroxide can be used to treat:

- *Heart and blood vessel diseases,* including angina pectoris; irregular heartbeat; stroke; peripheral vascular diseases such
  as Raynaud's phenomenon (interrupted circulation to the
  extremities), and gangrene of the fingers and toes; and vascular and cluster headaches.

- *Lung diseases,* including chronic obstructive pulmonary disease; emphysema; asthma; chronic bronchitis; bronchiecta-
  sis (a long-term degeneration of the bronchial tubes), and

pneumonia, including that caused by *Pneumocystis carinii* (a fungus that produces an AIDS-related pneumonia).

- *Infectious diseases*, including influenza, herpes zoster (shingles), herpes simplex (fever blister), systemic chronic candidiasis (yeast syndrome), Epstein-Barr virus (chronic fatigue syndrome), AIDS, chronic unresponsive bacterial infections, and parasitic infections.

- *Immune disorders*, including multiple sclerosis, rheumatoid arthritis, and hypersensitivity (allergy to a wide variety of environmental factors; see Chapter 3).

- *Miscellaneous conditions*, including a form of diabetes known as NIDDM (see page 84), parkinsonism (a group of nervous disorders), Alzheimer's disease, migraine headaches, chronic pain syndrome, metastatic cancer pain, and blood and lymph node cancers.

Usually, bio-oxidative therapy uses a very weak hydrogen peroxide solution of 0.0375 percent or less mixed into sugar or salt water, the same fluid base used for intravenous feeding in hospitals. The solution is administered in doses ranging from 50 to 500 milliliters (ml) as an intravenous drip into a vein. This dose is delivered over a period of from one to three hours. The treatment is painless except for the initial placement of the needle in the vein.

Treatments are normally given once a week for chronic illnesses, but can be given daily if the patient has an acute illness, such as pneumonia or influenza. Between five to twenty treatments are administered, depending on the patient's condition and the nature of the illness.

One to three months after treatment, the patient is checked to evaluate how well the treatment has worked and to determine if additional therapy is indicated. Some people, especially those with chronic illnesses, may need a series of five to ten additional infusions. Occasionally, chronically ill patients require maintenance therapy on a regular monthly schedule. As many as 100 treatments have been administered to some individuals, with no complications.

Over the past fifty years, thousands of patients have received intravenous hydrogen peroxide without any serious side effects. When this treatment was first administered, there was the rare problem of irritation in the vein being used. However, this was eliminated after the concentration and the rate of infusion were lowered.

Why is such an effective treatment with such minor side effects not administered more often? As was the case with many other effective treatments, intravenous hydrogen peroxide fell into disuse with the advent of antibiotics in the 1940s. Since then, few doctors have made the effort to learn about the latest in hydrogen peroxide research.

William Campbell Douglass, M.D., of Clayton, Georgia, has written about bio-oxidative therapy. (For more information on Dr. Douglass's book, see *Hydrogen Peroxide* in Appendix A.) Douglass, who is no longer in active practice, had one patient, a former heavy smoker named Roger, who had terminal emphysema. Roger was wheelchair-bound, and on a steady supply of oxygen. Nevertheless, his lips were always blue, and he was forced to sleep propped up because he was unable to breathe otherwise. According to Douglass,

> About ten minutes into the intravenous hydrogen peroxide treatment, Roger began to cough, indicating his lungs were already starting to clear. When he returned days later for the second treatment, I hardly recognized him! He looked so much better. . . . After his third treatment, he experienced some difficulty breathing. We reduced his concentration of intravenous hydrogen peroxide by half, and he felt no further adverse reaction.
>
> After four treatments, he discarded his wheelchair and stopped using the nasal oxygen. His face became pink, his appetite returned with a vengeance, and he rapidly gained eight pounds. And he sleeps flat as a board now—with no difficulty whatsoever. Any physician worth his salt would be amazed at this kind of recovery. Improvement like this is simply unheard of in emphysema patients.[7]

Other doctors have also had very good results. The late Stephen K. Elsasser, D.O., of Metamora, Illinois, gave intravenous hydrogen peroxide for correction of chronic candidiasis, or yeast syndrome. He found that such patients often had viral infections, and that treatments with intravenous hydrogen peroxide brought relief. He also used it for people with chronic bronchitis. Dr. Elsasser's patients did not experience side effects.[8]

Kirk Morgan, M.D., of Louisville, Kentucky, administered intravenous hydrogen peroxide to assist a patient with genital herpes. The patient, a man in his late thirties, used to suffer frequent, severe rashes. Now, the patient has only some slight redness that appears every once in a while.

Annette Stoesser, M.D., of Roswell, New Mexico, said, "The first time I ever used intravenous hydrogen peroxide was on myself to get rid of a bad cold. . . . The next morning . . . [i]t felt like there never had been anything wrong with me." She also used the treatment on a patient who had shingles, with good results. Dr. Stoesser finds bio-oxidative therapy to be most helpful for people with emphysema: "With hydrogen peroxide treatment, they feel better and need to use much less oxygen to help in breathing."

People with severe chronic illnesses, such as heart disease or emphysema, often find themselves dependent on drugs and tethered to machines. Intravenous hydrogen peroxide, a safe, simple, near-painless therapy, could give such patients hope for a better quality of life if it was employed more widely. In the next chapter, we will look at a supplement that may hold the key to prolonged life.

Chapter 16

Combating the Effects of Age With DHEA

Every minute of every day, numerous chemical reactions occur within our bodies. These reactions are controlled by substances called *hormones*. Most people know about testosterone and estrogen, the sex hormones, and adrenaline, a hormone that increases the heart rate. However, these are just a few of the hundreds of hormones produced by the body.

One of these hormones is dehydroepiandrosterone (DHEA). Research has shown that DHEA is an important factor in a number of bodily functions pertaining to health and longevity. Research has also shown that the amount of DHEA produced by the body declines with age, and that DHEA replacement therapy may help counteract some of the degenerative diseases that occur more frequently as people grow older.

In this chapter, we will first discuss DHEA's effects within the body. We will then see how DHEA can be used to help the body resist age.

HOW DHEA AFFECTS THE BODY

DHEA is produced by the adrenal glands, which sit on top of the kidneys. It is the most abundant hormone in the bloodstream. The body uses some of its DHEA supply to create testosterone, the primary male sex hormone, and estrogen, the primary female sex hormone. The exact amounts made depend on an individual's sex, age, and medical condition. Some DHEA becomes corticosterone, another hormone. (This is why DHEA is sometimes called "the mother of all hormones.") Some DHEA is also used to create DHEA-sulfate, or DHEAS. DHEA is quickly cleared from the bloodstream via the kidneys, while DHEAS remains in the blood for a longer period of time. (For more information on DHEA, see *DHEA* in Appendix A.)

DHEA production increases rapidly once a person reaches puberty. It peaks in one's twenties, and declines thereafter. It is estimated that by age seventy, production declines by about 75 percent.[1,2] Of course, each individual is different, and some people maintain relatively high DHEA levels even as they age.

Researchers think that DHEA affects the body in several ways:

- *It can help improve memory and mood.* People who have taken DHEA have reported that they sleep better, can remember things more easily, and have an enhanced sense of well-being. In one study, DHEA helped older people who suffered from depression.[3] A second study showed that patients with Alzheimer's disease had 48 percent less DHEA in their bloodstreams than other people in the same age group.[4]

- *It can help thin the blood and reduce cholesterol levels.* Blood that is too thick is prone to clotting. These clots can become trapped in the coronary arteries and produce heart attacks. There is some evidence that DHEA can help thin the blood.[5] Animal studies indicate that DHEA also helps reduce cholesterol levels, which can keep fatty deposits from building up on artery walls.[6,7] In addition, doctors have found that DHEAS levels are lower in men with a history of heart disease than in men with no such history.[8] However, more studies are needed in this area before we fully understand the link between DHEA and heart health.

- *It helps strengthen and normalize the immune system.* As the body ages, its resistance to infection often declines. DHEA has been shown to bolster the immune system in both animals and humans.[9,10] It also improves the effectiveness of vaccinations in older people.[11] In addition, DHEA is a valuable indicator of disease. In one study, women who developed breast cancer had lower-than-normal amounts of DHEA byproducts in their urine as long as nine years before the cancer developed.[12] Research also indicates that AIDS does not develop in people with HIV until DHEA levels start to drop.[13,14] In some people, the immune system creates problems by attacking the body itself in what is called an *autoimmune response*. This happens in lupus, an inflammatory condition that can affect the skin, blood vessels, kidneys, and nervous system. In one study, DHEA helped ten lupus patients.[15] Patients with other autoimmune diseases, such as rheumatoid arthritis, multiple sclerosis, and scleroderma, are often found to have low DHEA levels.

- *It helps prevent osteoporosis.* Postmenopausal women are especially prone to osteoporosis, in which the bones lose calcium and become brittle, because amounts of the female hormones estrogen and progesterone are reduced. Not surprisingly, DHEA levels in postmenopausal women are also reduced. Low levels of DHEA have been linked to reduced bone mass and the development of osteoporosis.[16,17]

- *It helps prevent diabetes.* Many people develop diabetes as they age. In diabetes, the body loses its ability to control levels of sugar in the blood. This occurs because insulin, which regulates blood sugar, becomes ineffective. DHEA has shown an ability to enhance insulin's effectiveness.[18–20]

- *It possibly encourages fat loss and muscle gain.* There is some evidence that DHEA decreases the percentage of body fat while increasing the percentage of muscle mass, apparently by speeding up the body's metabolism, or rate of energy usage. In one study, DHEA appeared to decrease both the size and number of fat cells in obese animals.[21] However, results so far have been inconclusive, and more studies are needed.

USING DHEA TO HELP THE BODY RESIST AGE

Some doctors think that DHEA may increase longevity. According to one theory, DHEA can switch on "youth" genes that are shut down when DHEA levels fall with age. It is also thought that falling DHEA levels upset the body's hormonal balance, which leads to various problems.[22] More research is needed in this area.

Much of the research that has been done on DHEA has been done on animals, and these studies have shown an increase in longevity. Such results may not be transferable to humans though, because rodents, unlike humans, have little DHEA circulating in their bloodstreams.[23,24]

Human DHEA research is in the early stages. Yet, one three-month study has indicated that supplemental DHEA can help both men and women. The people in this study, who were between the ages of forty and seventy, reported a greater sense of well-being after taking the supplements. They said they had more energy, were more relaxed, and slept better. Blood tests showed that their bloodstream DHEAS levels reached those found in young adults.[25]

DHEA does appear to affect men and women differently. For women, the issue is complicated by the fact that many older women receive hormone replacement therapy (HRT) to counteract menopausal symptoms such as hot flashes and night sweats. HRT is itself a complex topic that is beyond the scope of this book. We believe that women who are on HRT should discuss DHEA thoroughly with their health professionals.

Actually, anyone who wants to take DHEA should talk to his or her doctor before beginning a supplement program (see "Self-Medication and DHEA"). The use of DHEA is still controversial in medical circles. Some doctors believe that sup-

Self-Medication and DHEA

DHEA is available over the counter, and some people do self-medicate with DHEA. However, DHEA is still being tested in humans, so our knowledge of this hormone is incomplete. Also, it can worsen existing prostate problems, including prostate cancer, and can adversely affect women with reproductive-tract cancers. There is also a problem with the form of DHEA that is used. Many doctors believe that Mexican wild yam extract, a popular over-the-counter product, cannot increase DHEA levels in the body.

Therefore, we would urge you to *always* take DHEA under a doctor's care. Your health professional is familiar with your medical history, and can order blood and other tests to monitor your hormone levels.

plemental DHEA can reduce the amount of hormone made by the body itself. Others believe that high dosages can lead to liver damage. Still others think that supplemental DHEA cannot do much of anything.

Nevertheless, other doctors think that supplemental DHEA is a good idea for people who have low levels of DHEA to begin with. (This can be determined by a blood test or other laboratory procedure.) Dr. Kurk uses DHEA in his own practice, starting women on 10 mg a day and men on 25 mg a day. Most people who might be helped by DHEA are over age forty. It is very rare that DHEA would be recommended for someone under age thirty. Anyone who takes DHEA should be monitored by his or her doctor.

It is a good idea when taking DHEA to make sure you take supplemental antioxidants, such as vitamin C, vitamin E, and selenium. This can prevent against free-radical liver damage. (For more information on free radicals and antioxidants, see Chapters 1, 6, and 7.) You may also want to ask your doctor about using pregnenolone, DHEA's hormonal precursor (see *Pregnenolone* in Appendix A).

DHEA is a promising new weapon in the antiaging arsenal because it is involved in vital functions throughout the body. Even so, more research is needed on this fascinating and important hormone. In the meantime, see your doctor if you think DHEA might help you. In the next chapter, we'll discuss another antiaging formula called Gerovital.

Chapter 17

The Gerovital Secret of Long Life

Aging starts and ends in each of the body's individual cells. As time passes, cellular regeneration slows down while cellular degeneration speeds up. A delay in the process of growing old would occur if we could stop, or at least defer, the deterioration in this most basic of bodily units. Or, perhaps, we might be able to rejuvenate whatever youthfulness remains in the cells. However we approach the problem, we could discover the secret of long life if we could learn how to control age at the cellular level.

Such an antiaging substance has already been created. It contains an anesthetic used in dental offices throughout the world. The substance causes cellular aging to slow down markedly, so that the person who receives it can live a full natural life span. This substance is called Gerovital.

In this chapter, we will first see what the full potential human life span actually is by examining an Ecuadorian village where people routinely live to be more than 100 years old. We will then discuss Gerovital—what it is, what it does, and how it can help you live as long a life as possible.

THE HUMAN LIFE SPAN CAN BE EXTENDED

According to researchers and gerontologists, the human life span depends on two critical factors. One is the average life expectancy of the individual cells. The other is the genetically predetermined number of times each of those cells can divide. For instance, it has been shown that cells have an average life expectancy of two years. If a cell has a genetically predetermined potential to divide sixty times, then it will live a total of 120 years. Indeed, scientists have determined that the human life span under ideal conditions is 120 years.

This figure is derived from observations of relatively long-lived peoples who live in three regions of the world: in an isolated area of Pakistan known as Hunzaland; in the highlands of Georgia, a country that used to be part of the old Soviet Union; and in the village of Vilcabamba in southern Ecuador. All three areas are mountainous and remote, and all three have been relatively untouched by modern life.

Dr. Walker visited Vilcabamba in 1981 as part of a scientific expedition. About 15 percent of the village's 814 people were over ninety years old. At least fourteen were over 100, including a 132-year-old man who was the oldest person in the Western Hemisphere. These people were full of energy and vigor, even at such advanced ages. Degenerative diseases, such as atherosclerosis, diabetes, cancer, and Alzheimer's disease, were unknown to them. Generally, they died when their bodies simply wore out, with little decline in function beforehand. What was their secret?

To learn the answer, Dr. Walker took hair samples from fifty Vilcabambans. Forty were elderly, and seven were more than 100 years old. When these samples were analyzed, it was found that the mineral balance in the hair exactly matched the mineral balance in the diet. The Vilcabambans were made up of exactly what they ate and drank. Dr. Walker and others concluded that the Vilcabambans lived to ripe old ages because they ate and drank pure food and water, and led generally healthy lives.[1]

It helped that the Vilcabambans were exposed to very little pollution. There were fewer than twenty cars in the area, and practically no industry. There was no need for exercise as such, since most of the people worked on unmechanized farms high on the hillsides. This made them very physically fit.

The Vilcabamban diet consisted almost entirely of fresh fruits and vegetables, either farm-raised or picked from the wild. The people ate little meat, and kept chickens only for the eggs. There were no canned or prepared foods, and no refrigeration. Thus, food had to be eaten fresh, and often was eaten raw.

Interestingly, the Vilcabambans did smoke tobacco and drink alcohol. But the tobacco was cured without any additives and was made into leaf-wrapped cigars, not paper-wrapped cigarettes. The local drink was a fiery grain alcohol called *aquadiente*, and may have served to protect the residents against foodborne disease organisms.

The water seemed to be especially healthful, as it contained the perfect balance of minerals needed for longevity. These minerals included, among others, calcium, magnesium, selenium, and zinc (see Chapters 5 and 6). Selenium is an important antioxidant. Magnesium helps protect the heart. Calcium, along with other minerals, helps to regulate the heartbeat.

There are many aspects of life in Vilcabamba that would be difficult to duplicate in an industrialized society. (For more information on this remarkable village, see *Secrets of Long Life* in Appendix A.) However, it is important to remember that many ailments, including heart disease and several forms of cancer, are linked to diet and lifestyle. Indeed, like the Vilcabambans, all people really are what they put into their bodies as food and drink. Unfortunately, many people in the United States have poor diets, which when combined with a lack of exercise and an overload of stress, rob them of their health. That is why there is only one person over 100 years of age for every 1.7 million people in the United States, while there is one centenarian for every 58 people in Vilcabamba.[2]

GEROVITAL AND THE ANTIAGING EFFECT

One person who believed strongly in the benefits of a healthy diet was Professor Ana Aslan, M.D., Ph.D., director of the National Institute of Gerontologic Research and Geriatric Medicine in Bucharest, Rumania. Before her death in 1988 at the age of ninety-one, Dr. Aslan had become famous as the developer of an injectable formula based on components of procaine, a dental anesthetic. This formula, which she named Gerovital, was found to have remarkable antiaging properties, properties that could help reverse the effects of living in a modern, industrialized society.

The institute attracted the attention of such political notables as John Kennedy, Indira Gandhi, Charles de Gaulle, Mao Tse-tung, Nikita Khruschev, Leonid Brezhnev, Konrad Adenauer, Marshal Tito, and Ho Chi Minh. Actors Marlene Dietrich, Lillian Gish, Charlie Chaplin, and Kirk Douglas, and artists Pablo Picasso and Salvador Dali, also went there. All received Gerovital therapy.

Exactly what is Gerovital? It consists of the local anesthetic procaine hydrochloride, commonly used by dentists and podiatrists, mixed with buffering agents and other substances. The additives transform the anesthetic into a new formula that helps reverse the aging process. There are several different formulations of Gerovital.

Gerovital has helped Dr. Kurk's own patients. Over the years, people had hobbled into his Long Island office complaining of arthritis. Conventional therapies, such as cortisone injections in the affected joint, provided only temporary relief. He then read an article about Dr. Aslan and her use of a procaine-based formula called Gerovital. Dr. Kurk started using plain procaine on his arthritic patients. He noticed that not only did the procaine relieve the joint pain, but that his patients looked better, too. They seemed more relaxed and less haggard.

During the ensuing months, as Dr. Kurk continued to give procaine injections, some male patients began to comment on how their sex lives had improved, and how they felt greater energy and less fatigue. Female patients reported that they had fewer leg cramps while walking, and fewer night cramps. They said they felt sexier and younger as well. It was at that point that Dr. Kurk decided to contact Dr. Aslan for more information. If plain procaine could provide such benefits, what might Gerovital do?

Unfortunately, Dr. Kurk learned that Gerovital cannot be legally imported into the United States because the U.S. Food and Drug Administration (FDA) has not approved of its use. This frustrated both Dr. Kurk and Dr. Aslan, since plain procaine was a poor substitute for Gerovital.

As a result, in 1977, the Rumanian government invited Dr. Kurk to Bucharest so he could study with Dr. Aslan and work alongside her large team of physicians, biochemists, pharmacists, biologists, and other scientists. He learned how to prepare and administer Gerovital, and he participated in studies that measured the effects of Gerovital upon aging populations. He also talked to some of the patients who were living at the institute as paid volunteer test subjects. Some were ninety or older, and looking remarkably well and alert for their ages. These people walked briskly and strongly, and their skin was relatively free of wrinkles. The therapy had few if any side effects.

How does Gerovital work? Dr. Aslan believed that as part of the aging process, the body loses its ability to replace worn-out cells. As cells age, they become less flexible, which reduces their ability to function. Red blood cells are especially affected by a loss of flexibility, because flexibility allows them to pass more easily through capillaries, the tiny blood vessels that connect arteries to veins. Gerovital helps promote the production of new cells, which helps the body rejuvenate itself.[3]

Gerovital is broken down into a number of components within the body. One of those components is activated ethanolamine. This substance helps form phospholipids, the fat-based chemicals that are incorporated into the membranes of red blood cells. Phospholipids determine how flexible the cells will be.

Experiments have shown that in older people, Gerovital makes aging, inflexible red blood cells become as elastic as those of young people. When exposed to Gerovital, other body cells also contain greater amounts of energy and produce larger quantities of nutrients.

Gerovital can reduce pain, relax the blood vessels, counteract spasms, and affect the nervous system. It has been used to treat the following problems:

- Lessened energy and lack of vitality

- Nervous system disorders, including diminished hearing ability, reduced visual acuity, and dulled mental functions, such as memory loss

- Muscle and joint difficulties, especially tendonitis, arthritis, and rheumatism

- Skin problems, including baldness, psoriasis, and wrinkles

- Cardiovascular problems, such as high cholesterol levels, angina pectoris, and varicose veins

- Disorders of the gastrointestinal system, such as intestinal ulcers and stomach distress

Gerovital has shown an ability to minimize the feeling of illness in a sick person, and to give that person an increased capacity for physical and mental activity. Additionally, it improves muscle tone, the cardiovascular reaction to stress, and the body's use of oxygen. It may help restore use of the limbs to those suffering from stroke. It fights depression. Electroencephalographs, or brain-wave graphs, of depressed people show significant improvement when Gerovital is administered.

Dr. Aslan and her Rumanian colleagues, and others, have published their findings in scientific journals.[4-16] However, no full-scale studies have been published in this country. It is important to remember that Gerovital does not come from a drug company. It is very easily made in a doctor's office, which means it is not worth patenting. Therefore, it is simply not worth the millions of dollars that full-scale testing would require.

As a result, the use of Gerovital in the United States is still a controversial matter among doctors. Some doctors insist that too few studies been done with this substance, and those that have been done are of poor design. Many of these doctors do not believe that Gerovital works at all.[17] However, wholistic doctors such as Dr. Kurk do not rely on studies as much as conventional doctors do. Instead, wholistic doctors tend to go by how well a particular treatment improves the condition of their patients.

For people over seventy-five years of age, the course of treatment consists of one five-milliliter injection of Gerovital three times a week for four weeks. A second course of twelve to sixteen injections is given following a ten-day rest period. As many courses as a doctor deems necessary can be administered.

For people between the ages of thirty-five and seventy-four, a course of treatment to retard the aging process involves twelve to sixteen injections followed by a resting period of from one to two months. This is followed by another series of twelve to sixteen injections. This treatment may go on indefinitely to forestall the aging process.

A testing procedure is often used to insure that the patient will not have a bad reaction to Gerovital. The patient is administered a small quantity of solution in an injection under the skin. If the patient does not have a bad reaction to the small injection, another small injection is given into the muscle. If again the patient does not have a bad reaction, the full treatment may be given in complete safety. Gerovital can also be taken orally, but injections are preferable.

Most people's life spans fall far short of the 120-year life span that scientists believe is possible. However, the people of Vilcabamba provide living proof that it is not impossible to live not only a long life, but an active and vigorous one as well. If you want to live a longer and healthier life, there is no substitute for the basics of proper diet, proper exercise, and proper rest. But Gerovital can reverse some of the effects of age, and help you live as full a life as possible. In the next chapter, we'll see how you can put together a total long-life program.

Chapter 18

Creating Your Own Antiaging Program

There is an ancient saying, "We grow too soon old and too late smart." Our younger years are spent learning what life is all about. As we age, we become mature enough to really appreciate what we've learned. With the arrival of our middle years, though, our youthful vitality can start to deteriorate. Thus, we may lose the capacity to put what we've learned into practice. What's more, we believe that we can't do anything about it.

That belief, however, is false. We may not be able to stop the aging process, but we can certainly learn to retard and even reverse some of its effects. Wrinkles, fatigue, memory loss, arthritis, heart disease, cancer—none of these conditions is the inevitable result of aging. It is true that many degenerative diseases have a strong genetic component, and that genetics can well affect the rate at which each of us ages. Nevertheless, we cannot ignore the effects of lifestyle on disease and the aging process. In this chapter, we will see how you may put the information covered in this book to good use by creating an overall antiaging program. (For more information on various therapies and treatments, see *Prescription for Nutritional Healing* in Appendix A.)

STEP 1: EAT A HEALTHY DIET

Your diet should be based on organically grown fruits and vegetables, and lots of whole grains. You should reduce the amounts of meat, poultry, and dairy products (except for yogurt) you consume. You must also avoid junk foods, salt, sugar, and preservatives. You should drink bottled or filtered water, or herbal tea. Avoid tap water (even bottled tap water), alcohol, soda, coffee, or regular tea.

A healthy diet is the solid foundation of an antiaging program. That is because many of the degenerative diseases associated with age are caused, at least in part, by a poor diet. Too much salt can lead to high blood pressure. Too much fat and cholesterol can lead to atherosclerosis, in which fatty deposits form within the blood vessels. Both high blood pressure and atherosclerosis are major causes of heart disease and stroke. Excessive fat intake predisposes one to obesity, which is associated with both heart disease and cancer. Obesity is also associated with diabetes, as is excessive sugar intake. As we have seen, poor diet causes free radical production (Chapter 1), brain allergies (Chapter 3), and mineral imbalances (Chapter 4).

Eating a diet based on fruits, vegetables, and whole grains will allow you to avoid many of these pitfalls. Fresh fruits and vegetables contain abundant vitamins, minerals, and antioxidants, the substances that counteract free-radical damage. Whole grains contain a lot of fiber, which is important for intestinal health (see Chapter 10). High-fiber foods also fight obesity. As we saw in Chapter 12, yogurt is a wonderful high-protein food. However, other dairy foods, such as cheese and sour cream, contain a lot of fat, as do many types of meat. Furthermore, a diet that contains a lot of healthy ingredients can still be bad for you if those ingredients contain chemical residues. Organic produce may cost a little more, but it's worth it. (For more information on nutrition, see *Lick the Sugar Habit* and *Secrets of Living Fat-Free* in Appendix A.)

Just as important as what you eat is what you drink. Our list of recommended fluids is short, but with good reason. Tap water often contains harmful contaminants. Alcohol impairs mental functioning and can cause liver damage. It is also high in calories. Coffee and tea contain not only caffeine but other unhealthy substances. Soda is high in sugar (or sugar substitute), as is fruit juice. Even club soda is a problem because it may be made with impure water. Stick with purified water and herbal tea.

STEP 2: INCREASE YOUR EXERCISE, REDUCE YOUR STRESS

Start a regular exercise and stress-reduction program tailored to your physical and mental capabilities.

As we saw in Chapter 2, stress can cause the body to age faster than normal. (It can also lead people to seek relief in practices such as smoking, drinking, and drug use, which by themselves accelerate the aging process.) Exercise fights stress in two ways. First, it makes the body more fit, and thus counteracts the physical effects of stress. Second, exercise releases morphinelike chemicals called endorphins in the brain, and thus counteracts the psychological effects of stress. Exercise can also help fight obesity.

There are two forms of exercise. Aerobic exercise strengthens the heart and lungs, while anaerobic exercise strengthens the muscles and joints. The former includes walking and jogging, the latter involves weight training. Both are important for health. However, the most important part of any fitness program is the commitment to exercise. You are never too old to begin. On the contrary, the older you are, the more important fitness becomes.

Exercise is important, but you should still account for your physical limitations—forget the "no pain, no gain" idea. See your doctor before beginning any exercise program, especially if you have a pre-existing health condition. If you are out of shape, start slowly. Walking is an excellent exercise; some shopping malls open early so older walkers can exercise in comfort. Aqua aerobics, or exercises done in a pool, allow you to work out without straining arthritic or injured joints. There are also low-impact aerobics specifically designed for older adults (see *Prime Moves* in Appendix A). And don't forget the rebounding exercises mentioned in Chapter 11. They are not only good for digestion, but for overall fitness as well.

You can also fight stress with one of the other stress-reduction techniques discussed in Chapter 2, such as meditation or biofeedback. These methods produce the relaxation response, which is the direct opposite of the stress response, which causes your heart rate, blood pressure, and respiration rate to all increase. The relaxation response causes these functions to slow down, which allows the body to maintain and repair itself.

One popular, simple way to induce the relaxation response is called progressive relaxation. This involves forcefully contracting a set of muscles, such as those of the face, for one or two seconds and then letting them go. Start at either your head or your feet, and work your way up or down your body, tensing and relaxing one muscle group after another.

For more information on stress management, see *Feeling Good* and *The Complete Guide to Your Emotions & Your Health* in Appendix A. Or you can see what's being offered through the continuing education program at your local high school or college. Just be sure to speak to your doctor first if you are prone to problems such as anxiety or depression.

STEP 3: USE SUPPLEMENTS WISELY

Consider taking nutritional supplements both to support a healthy diet and to ease specific health problems.

Under ideal conditions, everyone would get the necessary vitamins and minerals from dietary sources alone. However, few people enjoy ideal conditions. Busy schedules often lead to skipped or rushed meals, which can over time lead to nutritional deficiencies. Pre-existing medical conditions often require additional nutrients. In addition, all of us are subjected to the pervasive effects of pollution in our water, air, and soil. These toxins can cause accelerated aging because they create harmful free radicals (see Chapters 1 and 7).

Table 17.1. Recommended Daily Vitamin and Mineral Amounts

Nutrient	Recommendation
Vitamin A and Beta-carotene[1]	25,000–50,000 International Units (IUs)
Vitamin D$_3$	100–400 IUs
Vitamin E	400 IUs
Thiamin (vitamin B$_1$)	100–300 mg
Riboflavin (vitamin B$_2$)	50–200 mg
Pyridoxine (vitamin B$_6$)	100–300 mg
Cobalamin (vitamin B$_{12}$)	25–100 mcg
Folic acid	800–1,000 mcg
Pantothenic acid	100–500 mg
Biotin	300 mcg
Manganese	5–10 mg
Iodine[2]	150–300 mcg
Potassium[3]	99 mcg

1. At least 50% of the dosage should be in the form of beta-carotene, the substance from which vitamin A is made within the body. Vitamin A by itself can be toxic at high dosages.

2. This dosage is for people who do not routinely eat iodized salt and/or seaweed products. If you eat these items regularly, you may not need iodine at all. See your doctor.

3. Potassium intake should be kept in a 1:1 ratio with sodium intake. Since most people consume too much sodium, we urge you to reduce your sodium intake in addition to taking supplemental potassium.

Therefore, you may want to add nutritional supplements to your antiaging program. We would urge you to speak to your doctor before beginning a supplement program, especially if you have a pre-existing medical condition, are exposed to strong sources of free radicals, or have symptoms that may suggest a nutritional deficiency. Your doctor will probably want to give you a basic physical, and may want to order a hair mineral analysis as well (see Chapter 4).

If you are in good health, you may just want to take a multivitamin/multimineral capsule every day. How much of each nutrient should you take? See Chapter 5 for information on the major minerals: calcium, phosphorus, and magnesium. See Chapter 6 for information on selenium and zinc, two of the important trace minerals. See Chapter 8 for information on niacin (vitamin B$_3$) and chromium. See Chapter 9 for information on vitamin C. Table 17.1 gives recommended amounts of other important vitamins and minerals.

You may want to add some supplements to those listed in the table. See Chapter 6 for information on germanium and iron, and Chapter 9 for information on vitamin C's bioflavonoid partner, OPC. See Chapter 13 for information on oral chelation.

STEP 4: WHEN YOU NEED SOMETHING MORE

From time to time, you may want to add other steps to your antiaging program. Some steps you can take on your own. Others require a doctor's supervision.

Over-the-Counter Remedies

If your bowels trouble you occasionally, use an internal cleanser. (If the problem is chronic, see your doctor or a gastroenterologist.) If you need additional energy, use herbal therapy.

Bowel problems are among the most common health complaints. This is not surprising, since many people eat diets that are poor in nutrients such as fiber, vitamins, and minerals, and rich in antinutrients such as sugar, salt, and excess fat. A poor diet can lead to the development of toxins within the digestive system. These toxins can harm the gut flora, the millions of tiny plants and animals that live in the intestines and help the body digest food. An imbalance in the gut flora can allow disease-producing organisms to flourish.

Even people who generally eat healthy diets can suffer the occasional bout of bowel trouble. Travel, periods of intense stress, and antibiotics can all affect the gut flora. If this happens to you, the internal cleansers discussed in Chapter 11 may bring relief.

If you suffer from chronic bowel trouble, you will want to see a gastroenterologist, a doctor who specializes in bowel disease. You may be surprised that we would recommend a visit to a conventional doctor. Keep in mind, though, that conventional medicine does have its strong points, and diagnosis is one of them. A proper diagnosis is important to any doctor, conventional or wholistic, because it is important to know exactly what is causing the problem. In some cases, such as acute appendicitis or bowel cancer, you may very well want to accept conventional treatment, such as surgery. However, the vast majority of bowel problems are not that acute and can be treated with less drastic methods.

Fatigue is another common health complaint. Again, it is important to see your doctor if you suffer from chronic fatigue. If he or she cannot find a specific cause, you may want to try one of the herbal remedies in Chapter 14.

Doctor-Prescribed Therapies

If you are suffering from a serious illness, such as heart disease, emphysema, or severe arthritis, consider seeing a doctor who specializes in alternative therapies, especially if conventional therapy hasn't worked for you. You may also want to see a wholistic doctor if you simply want to pursue your antiaging program more vigorously.

Millions of people worldwide live with chronic illnesses. For many of these people, conventional medicine has provided a near-normal existence, even prolonged life. However, the treatments used in conventional medicine can produce side effects. In some cases, they may not help certain patients.

Alternative treatments—including chelation therapy (Chapter 13), intravenous hydrogen peroxide (Chapter 14), DHEA (Chapter 16), and Gerovital (Chapter 17)—tend to be gentler than conventional medicine in their actions. This can reduce the number of side effects, or can eliminate side effects altogether. Such alternative treatments can still be very effective, despite their gentleness. Talk to a wholistic doctor about using these therapies, either to treat a specific problem or as part of a general antiaging program.

In this book, we have discussed various supplements and treatments, and how they can help prolong life. These supplements and treatments are good ways of both preventing and fighting the diseases associated with age. However, they are no substitute for a proper diet, along with proper exercise and proper rest. Put all these elements together into your own antiaging program, and maybe you can live a century or more. But even if you do not, you will look better, feel healthier, and have the energy to do the things you really want to do in life. And isn't that the greatest fountain of youth there is?

Appendix A

Suggested Reading Materials

Chelation therapy study. American College for Advancement in Medicine (ACAM), Executive Director Edward Shaw, 23121 Verdugo Drive, Laguna Hills CA 92653, 1-800-532-3688 or 714-583-7666.

The Chelation Way. Morton Walker. Avery Publishing Group, 120 Old Broadway, Garden City Park NY 11040, 1-800-548-5757, 1990.

The Complete Guide to Your Emotions & Your Health. Emrika Padus and the Editors of *Prevention* Magazine. Rodale Press, Emmaus PA, 1986.

DHEA: A Practical Guide. Ray Sahelian. Avery Publishing Group, 120 Old Broadway, Garden City Park NY 11040, 1-800-548-5757, 1996.

Feeling Good: The New Mood Therapy. David D. Burns. William Morrow and Company, New York, 1980.

The Ginger Book. Stephen Fulder. Avery Publishing Group, 120 Old Broadway, Garden City Park NY 11040, 1-800-548-5757, 1996.

The Ginseng Book. Stephen Fulder. Avery Publishing Group, 120 Old Broadway, Garden City Park NY 11040, 1-800-548-5757, 1996.

The Healing Powers of Elderberry Internal Cleansing. Morton Walker. New Way of Life, Inc., 485 High Ridge Road, Stamford CT 06905, 203-322-1551.

Hydrogen Peroxide: Medical Miracle. William Campbell Douglass. Second Opinion Publishing, P.O. Box 467939, Atlanta GA 30346-7939, 1-800-728-2288.

Jumping for Health. Morton Walker. Avery Publishing Group, 120 Old Broadway, Garden City Park NY 11040, 1-800-548-5757, 1989.

Lick the Sugar Habit. Nancy Appleton. Avery Publishing Group, 120 Old Broadway, Garden City Park NY 11040, 1-800-548-5757, 1996.

Pregnenolone: Nature's Feel Good Hormone. Ray Sahelian. Avery Publishing Group, 120 Old Broadway, Garden City Park NY 11040, 1-800-548-5757, 1997.

Prescription for Nutritional Healing. James F. Balch and Phyllis A. Balch. 2nd ed. Avery Publishing Group, 120 Old Broadway, Garden City Park NY 11040, 1-800-548-5757, 1997.

Prime Moves: Low Impact Exercises for the Mature Adult. Diane Edwards with Kathy Nash. Avery Publishing Group, 120 Old Broadway, Garden City Park NY 11040, 1-800-548-5757, 1992.

Secrets of Living Fat-Free. Sandra Woodruff. Avery Publishing Group, 120 Old Broadway, Garden City Park NY 11040, 1-800-548-5757, 1997.

Secrets of Long Life. Morton Walker. Freelance Publications, 484 High Ridge Road, Stamford CT 06905-3020, 203-322-1551, 1983.

Toxic Metal Syndrome: How Heavy Metal Poisons Can Affect Your Brain. H. Richard Casdorph and Morton Walker. Avery Publishing Group, 120 Old Broadway, Garden City Park NY 11040, 1-800-548-5757, 1995.

The Yeast Syndrome. John Parks Trowbridge and Morton Walker. Bantam Books, c/o Freelance Communications, 484 High Ridge Road, Stamford, CT 06905-3020, 203-322-1551, 1986.

Appendix B

Sources of Products and Services

Bio-Oxidative Therapy (intravenous hydrogen peroxide)

International Bio-Oxidative Medicine (IBOM) Foundation
Executive Director Suzanne R. Moore
P.O. Box 13205
Oklahoma City OK 73113-1205
405-478-4266

Chelation Therapy

American College for Advancement in Medicine (ACAM)
Executive Director Edward Shaw
23121 Verdugo Drive
Laguna Hills CA 92653
1-800-532-3688/714-583-7666

Elderberry Internal Cleansing

L & H Vitamins Inc.
37-10 Crescent Street
Long Island City NY 11101
1-800-221-1152/fax 718-361-1437

Germanium

DaVinci Laboratories
800-451-5190

Herbal Medicine

Golden State Herb Research Inc.
P.O. Box 810
Occidental CA 95465

Haussmann's Pharmacy
534-536 West Girard Avenue
Philadelphia PA 19123

Indiana Botanic Gardens Inc.
P.O. Box 5
Hammond IN 46325

K.D. Distributor Ltd.
1038 South Grand Avenue
Los Angeles CA 90015

Kwan Yin Herb Company
P.O. Box 18617
Spokane WA 99208

Nature's Herb Company
281 Ellis Street
San Francisco CA 94102

Penn Herb Company
603 North Second Street
Philadelphia PA 19123

Starwest Botanicals Inc.
11253 Trade Center Drive
Rancho Cordova CA 95742
916-853-9354/fax 916-853-9673

OPC

Primary Source
1916 Post Road, Second Floor
Fairfield CT 06430
1-888-666-1188, 203-256-1188/fax 203-255-9402

Parasitology

Great Smokies Diagnostic Laboratory
Laboratory Director Martin J. Lee, President Stephen Barrie
63 Zillicoa Street
Asheville NC 28801-1074
1-800-522-4762, 704-253-0621/fax 704-253-1127
E-mail: cs@gsdl.com

Rebounding devices

Nedak Manufacturing
President Bob Sanders, Sales Director Ken Seeley
120 West Douglas
O'Neill NE 68763
1-800-232-5762, 402-336-4083/fax 402-336-4941

Notes

Introduction

1. Walker M. *Secrets of Long Life.* Stamford CT: Freelance Publications, 1983, pp. 10–14.

Chapter 1
The Free Radical Reason for Premature Aging

1. Strehler B.L. *Aging: Some Social and Biological Aspects.* Washington DC: American Association for the Advancement of Science, 1960, p. 273.

2. Green M. Aging and disease. *Journal of Clinical Endocrinology and Metabolism* 10:207–228, 1981.

3. Harman D. Free radical theory of aging: the "free radical" diseases. *Age* 7:111–131, 1984.

4. Harman D. Prolongation of the normal life span by radiation protection chemicals. *Journal of Gerontology* 12:257–263, 1957.

5. Ames B.N. Dietary Carcinogens and anticarcinogens—oxygen radicals and degenerative diseases. *Science* 221:1256–1264, 1983.

6. Tappel A. On antioxidant nutrients—how they may protect

you from smog and other environmental pollutants and some aging reactions. *Executive Health* 16(6), March 1980.

7. Harman D. Aging: A theory based on free radical and radiation chemistry. *Journal of Gerontology* 11:298–300, 1956.

8. Harman D. Free radical theory of aging: the "free radical" diseases. *Age* 7:111–131, 1984.

9. Lubrano R. and others. Relationship between red blood cell lipid peroxidation, plasma hemoglobin, and red blood cell osmotic resistance before and after vitamin E supplementation in hemodialysis patients. *Artificial Organs* 10:245–250, 1986.

10. Pritchard K. and others. Triglyceride-lowering effect of dietary vitamin E in streptozocin-induced diabetic rats. *Diabetes* 35:278–281, 1986.

11. Kay M. and others. Oxidation as a possible mechanism of cellular aging: vitamin E deficiency causes premature aging and IgG binding to erythrocytes. *Proceedings of the National Academy of Science* 83:2463–2467, 1986.

12. Kent S. Solving the riddle of lipofuscin's origin may uncover clues to the aging process. *Geriatrics* 31:128–137, 1976.

13. Katz M. and others. Lipofuscin accumulation resulting from senescence and vitamin E deficiency: spectral properties and tissue distribution. *Mechanism of Aging and Development* 25:149–159, 1984.

14. Kishnamurthy S. The intriguing biological role of vitamin E. *Journal of Chem Ed* 60:465–467, 1983.

15. Katz M. and others. Lipofuscin accumulation resulting from senescence and vitamin E deficiency: spectral properties and tissue distribution. *Mechanism of Aging and Development* 25:149–159, 1984.

16. Burton G.W. and others. First proof that vitamin E is major lipid-soluble, chain-breaking antioxidant in human blood plasma. *Lancet* 2(8293):327, 1982.

17. Csallany A.S. and others. Effect of selenite, vitamin E, and N,N1-Diphenyl-pPhenylenediamine on liver organic solvent-

soluble lipofuscin pigments in mice. *Journal of Nutrition* 114: 1582–1587, 1984.

18. Burton G.W. and others. First proof that vitamin E is major lipid-soluble, chain-breaking antioxidant in human blood plasma. *Lancet* 2(8293):327, 1982.

19. Tappel A. Will antioxidant nutrients slow aging processes? *Geriatrics* 23:97–105, 1968.

20. Porta E. and others. Effects of the type of dietary fat at two levels of vitamin E in Wistar male rats during development and aging. Life span, serum biochemical parameters and pathological changes. *Mechanisms of Aging and Development* 13: 1–39, 1980.

21. Meydani M. and others. Effect of vitamin E, selenium, and age on lipid peroxidation events in rat cerebrum. *Nutrition Research* 5:1227–1236, 1985.

22. Meydani M. and others. Effect of vitamin E, selenium, and age on lipid peroxidation events in rat cerebrum. *Nutrition Research* 5:1227–1236, 1985.

23. Tufts University, Office of Communications. Vitamin E may help slow aging, Tufts nutritionists find. *Journal of the American Dietetic Association* 86:200, 1986.

24. Wartanowicz M. and others. The effect of alpha-tocopherol and ascorbic acid on the serum lipid peroxide level in elderly people. *Annals of Nutrition and Metabolism* 28:186–191, 1984.

25. Tolonen M. and others. Vitamin E and selenium supplementation in geriatric patients. *Biological Trace Element Research* 7:161–168, 1985.

26. Harman D. Free radical theory of aging: the "free radical" diseases. *Age* 7:111–131, 1984.

27. Tappel A. On antioxidant nutrients—how they may protect you from smog and other environmental pollutants and some aging reactions. *Executive Health* 16(6), March 1980.

Chapter 2
Stress as a Source of Premature Aging

1. Greenspan K. Nonpharmacologic approaches to stress management. *The Consequences of Stress: The Medical and Social Implications of Prescribing Tranquilizers.* A live televised symposium. New York City: Cornell University, 21 March 1979.

2. Selye H. What is stress? *The Second International Symposium on the Management of Stress.* Beverly Hills CA: International Health Resorts, Inc., 1986.

3. Selye H. What is stress? *The Second International Symposium on the Management of Stress.* Beverly Hills CA: International Health Resorts, Inc., 1986.

4. Selye H. What is stress? *The Second International Symposium on the Management of Stress.* Beverly Hills CA: International Health Resorts, Inc., 1986.

5. Editorial. *Journal of the American Medical Association* 3 October 1977.

Chapter 3
Brain Allergies and Premature Aging

1. Stavish G.E. and Stavish P.C. Mental illness: an allergic response. *Health Express,* March 1983, pp. 50, 67, 75.

2. Philpott W.H. and Kalita D.K. *Brain Allergies: The Psychonutrient Connection.* New Canaan CT: Keats Publishing, Inc., 1980, pp. 23–24.

3. Schmeck H.M. Addict's brain: chemistry holds hope for answers. *The New York Times,* Science Times, 25 January 1983, pp. C1, C6.

4. Michael Russell, telephone interview by Morton Walker.

5. Philpott W.H. and Kalita D.K. *Brain Allergies: The Psychonutrient Connection.* New Canaan CT: Keats Publishing, Inc., 1980, p. 7.

6. Philpott W.H. and Kalita D.K. *Brain Allergies: The Psy-*

chonutrient Connection. New Canaan CT: Keats Publishing, Inc., 1980, p. 16.

Chapter 4
Hair Mineral Analysis and Premature Aging

1. Lazar P. Hair analysis: what does it tell us? *Journal of the American Medical Association* 229:1908, 1974.

2. Ashmead W.D. *Chelated Mineral Nutrition*. Huntington Beach CA: International Institute of Natural Health Sciences, Inc., 1981, pp. 33–44.

3. Schrotenboer G. Hair analysis: what does it tell us? *Journal of the American Dental Association* 92:1214, 1974.

4. Laker M. On Determining Trace Element Levels in Man: The Uses of Blood and Hair. Reprinted from *Lancet*, 31 July 1982.

5. Kennington G.S. Soluble and fixed elements in mammalian hair. *Science* 155:588, 1967.

6. Shroeder H.A. and Nelson A.P. Trace metals in human hair. *Journal of Investigative Dermatology* 53:71, 1969.

7. Gershoff S., McGandy R., Nondastuda A., Pisdyabutra U., and Tantiwonge P. Trace minerals in human and rat hair. *American Journal of Clinical Nutrition* 30:868, 1977.

8. Fassel V.A. Quantitative element analyses by plasma emission spectroscopy. *Science* 202:183, 1978.

9. Habidge K.M., Walravens P.A., Brown R.M., Webster J., White S., Anthony M., and Roth R.L. Zinc nutrition of preschool children in the Denver Head Start program. *American Journal of Clinical Nutrition* 29:734, 1976.

10. Balch J.F. and Balch P.A. *Prescription for Nutritional Healing*. 2nd ed. Garden City Park NY: Avery Publishing Group, 1997, p. 26.

11. Cartwright G.E. and Wintrobe M.M. Copper metabolism in normal subjects. *American Journal of Clinical Nutrition* 14:224, 1964.

12. Jacob R., Klevay L., and Logan G. Hair as a biopsy material: index of hepatic metal; copper and zinc. *American Journal of Clinical Nutrition* 31:477, 1978.

13. Wintrobe M.M., Cartwright G.E., and Gubler C.J. Studies on the function and metabolism of copper. *American Journal of Clinical Nutrition* 50:395, 1953.

14. Deeming S. and Weber C. Hair analysis of trace elements in human subjects as influenced by age, sex, and contraceptive drugs. *American Journal of Clinical Nutrition* 31:1175, 1978.

Chapter 5
Minerals and Health: The Major Minerals

1. Marvelous minerals—Part 1. *Clearwater Natural News* II(2):1, October 1991.

2. Wade C. *Magic Minerals: Key to Better Health.* Nyack NY: Parker Publishing Co., 1967, pp. 4–5.

3. Clark L. *A Handbook of Natural Remedies for Common Ailments.* New York: Pocket Books, 1977.

4. Wade C. *Magic Minerals: Key to Better Health.* Nyack NY: Parker Publishing Co., 1967, pp. 93–101.

5. Hoffer A. and Walker M. *Putting It All Together: The New Orthomolecular Nutrition.* New Canaan CT: Keats Publishing, 1996, pp. 134, 140–141.

6. Hoffer A. and Walker M. *Putting It All Together: The New Orthomolecular Nutrition.* New Canaan CT: Keats Publishing, 1996, pp. 134, 140–141.

Chapter 6
Minerals and Health: The Trace Minerals

1. Kidd P.M. Germanium-132 (Ge-132): homeostatic normalizer and immunostimulant, a review of its preventive and therapeutic efficacy. *International Clinical Nutrition Review* 7:11–20, 1987.

2. Kidd P.M. Germanium-132 (Ge-132): homeostatic normalizer and immunostimulant, a review of its preventive and therapeutic efficacy. *International Clinical Nutrition Review* 7:11–20, 1987.

3. Anderson J. Paper read at the 21 February 1987 annual meeting of the Orthomolecular Medical Society.

4. Kirn T.F. Do low levels of iron affect body's ability to regulate temperature experience cold? *Journal of the American Medical Association* 260:607, 1988.

6. Schubert E.G. and Schilcher H. Modern treatment of iron deficiency. *Private Hospitals, Clinics, and Sanitoria* 67:6, 1965.

Chapter 7
Stopping the Free Radical Attack With
Vitamins and Coenzyme Q10

1. Jacques P., Chylack L., McGandy R., and others. Antioxidant status in persons with and without senile cataract. *Archives of Ophthalmology* 106:337–340, 1988.

2. Airriess G., Changchit C., Chen L., and others. Increased vitamin E levels in the lungs of guinea pigs exposed to mainstream or sidestream smoke. *Nutrition Research* 8:653–661, 1988.

3. Hasselmark L., Malmgren R., Unge G., and others. Lowered platelet glutathione peroxidase activity in patients with intrinsic asthma. *Allergy* 45:523–527, 1990.

4. Barnes P. Reactive oxygen species and airway inflammation. *Free Radical Biomedicine* 9:235–243, 1990.

5. Jacques P., Chylack L., McGandy R., and others. Antioxidant status in persons with and without senile cataract. *Archives of Ophthalmology* 106:337–340, 1988.

6. Howard L. The neurological syndrome of vitamin E deficiency: laboratory and electrophysiologic assessment. *Nutritional Review* 48:169–177, 1990.

7. In K. Folkers and Y. Yamamura (eds): *Biomedical and Clin-*

ical Aspects of Coenzyme Q. Vol. 5. Amsterdam: Elsevier Science Publications BV, 1986, pp. 337–343.

8. *Clinical Endocrinology* 25:1019–1023, 1977.

9. *Journal of Adult Disease* 6:281–286, 1976.

10. *Current Therapeutic Research* 51:668–672, 1992.

11. *Communications in Chemistry, Pathology, and Pharmacology* 14:715, 1976.

12. *Research Communication in Chemistry, Pathology, and Pharmacology* 12:111, 1975.

13. Shiseta Y., Izumi K., and Abe H. Effect of coenzyme Q_7 treatment on blood sugar and ketone bodies of diabetics. *Journal of Vitaminology* 12:293, 1966.

14. Coenzyme Q. Presented at the American College of Nutrition Annual Meeting, San Francisco, 1996.

15. Therapy with coenzyme Q_{10} for muscular dystrophies and neurogenic atrophies. *Proceedings of The National Academy of Science*, 82:1513–1516, July 1985.

16. Vanfraechem J.H.P. and Folkers K. Coenzyme Q_{10} and physical performance. In Folkers K. and Yamamura Y. (eds): *Biomedical and Clinical Aspects of Coenzyme Q.* Vol. 3. Amsterdam: Elsevier/North Holland Biomedical Press, 1981, pp. 235–241.

17. *Journal of Molecular Medicine* 3:289–298, 1978.

18. In Folkers K. and Yamamura Y. (eds): *Biomedical and Clinical Aspects of Coenzyme Q.* Vol. 3. Amsterdam: Elsevier/North Holland Biomedical Press, 1981, pp. 339–412.

19. Kamikawa T. and others. Effects of coenzyme Q_{10} on exercise tolerance in chronic stable angina pectoris. *American Journal of Cardiology* 56:247, 1985.

20. Ishiyama T. and others. A clinical study of the effect of coenzyme Q on congestive heart failure. *Japanese Heart Journal* 17:32, 1976.

21. *Drug Experimental Clinical Research XI* 8:581–593, 1985.

22. Ishiyama T. and others. A clinical study of the effect of coenzyme Q on congestive heart failure. *Japanese Heart Journal* 17:32, 1976.

23. *Tohoku Journal of Experimental Medicine* 141(suppl):453–463, 1983.

24. In Lenaz G. (ed): *Coenzyme Q.* New York: John Wiley & Sons, 1985, pp. 479–505.

25. In Lenaz G. (ed): *Coenzyme Q Biochemistry, Bioenergetics, and Clinical Applications of Ubiquinone.* New York: Wiley-Interscience, 1985, pp. 479–507.

26. *Clinical Investigator* 71:S51–S54, 1993.

Chapter 8
Niacin: A Vitamin for Long Life

1. Goldsmith, G.A. The B vitamins: thiamin, riboflavin, niacin. In Breton G.H. and McHenry E.W. (eds): *Nutrition, A Comprehensive Treatise.* Vol. 2. New York: Academic Press, 1964, pp. 161–198.

2. Goldsmith G.A., Miller O.N., and Unglaub W.G. *Journal of Nutrition* 73:172–176, 1961.

3. Carlson L.A. and Oro L. *Acta Medica Scandinavica* 172:641–645, 1962.

4. Carlson, L.A. *Advances in Experimental Medicine and Biology* 4:327, 1969.

5. Ginoulhiac E., Tenconi L.T., and Chiancone F.M. 3-Pyridineacetic acid and nicotinic acid: blood levels, urinary elimination and excretion of nicotinic acid derivatives in man. *Nature* 193:948–949, 1962.

6. Meyers F.H., Jawetz E., and Goldfien A. *Review of Medical Pharmacology.* Los Altos CA: Lange Medical Publ, 1972, p. 118.

7. Carlson L.A. and Nye E.R. *Acta Medica Scandinavica* 1979:453, 1963.

8. Garg A. and Grundy S.M. Nicotinic acid as therapy for

dyslipidemia in non-insulin-dependent diabetes mellitus. *Journal of the American Medical Association.* 264(6): 723–726, 1990.

9. Anderson R.A. and Kozlovsky A.S. Chromium intake, absorption and excretion of subjects consuming self-selected diets. *American Journal of Clinical Nutrition* 41:1177–1183, 1985.

10. Anderson R.A. Chromium metabolism and its role in disease processes in man. *Clinical Physiology and Biochemistry* 4: 31–41, 1986.

11. Anderson R.A., Bryden N.A., and Polansky M.M. Dietary chromium intake. Freely chosen diets, institutional diets and individual foods. *Biological Trace Element Research* 32:117–121, 1992.

12. Urberg Martin. Screening for family dysfunction. *The Journal of Family Practice* 25(6):554, 556, 1987.

13. Gordon J.B. An easy and inexpensive way to lower cholesterol? *Western Journal of Medicine* 154:352, 1991.

Chapter 9
The Power of Vitamin C

1. Hoffer A. and Walker M. *Smart Nutrients: A Guide to Nutrients That Can Prevent and Reverse Senility* Garden City Park, NY: Avery Publishing Group, Inc., 1994, p. 144.

2. Bentrath A., Russuvan S., and Szent-Gyorgyi A. *Nature* 138:798, 1936.

3. Cojocaru A.F., Ruzieva R.H., Topaly E.E., and Topaly V.P. *Stud Biophys* 72:15, 1978.

4. Schneidewind E.M., Büge A., Kala H., Metzner J., and Zschumke A. Identifizierung eines aus Propolis isolierton antimikrobiell wirksamen Inheltsstoffes. *Pharmazie* 34:100, 1979.

5. Harborne J.B., Ingram J.L., King L., and Payne M. *Phytochemistry* 15:1485, 1976.

6. Pinkas J., Lavie D., and Charin M. *Phytochemistry* 7:169, 1968.

7. Shub T.A., Kagramanova K.A., Voropaeva S.D., and Kivmann G.Ia. Deistvie propolisa na shtammy zolotistogg stafilokokka, ustoichivye k antiotikam. *Antibiotiki* 26:268–271, 1981.

8. Rodale J.I. *The Health Seeker*. Emmaus PA: Rodale Books, 1957, p. 76.

9. Voelter, W. and Jung, G. *O-(2-Hydroxyethyl)-nitrosides. Experimental and Clinical Results*. Berlin: Springer, 1978.

10. Airola P. *Are You Confused?* Phoenix AZ: Health Plus, 1974, p. 161.

11. Havsteen B. Flavonoids, a class of natural products of high pharmacological potency. *Biochemical Pharmaceuticals* 32(7): 1141–1148, 1983.

12. Masquelier J. Pycnogenols: Recent advances in the therapeutic activity of procyanidins. *Journal of Medicinal Plant Research*, July 1980, pp. 243–256.

13. Murray M.T. *Encyclopedia of Nutritional Supplements*. Rocklin CA: Prima Publishing, 1996, p. 324.

14. *Zeitschrift fur Allgemeinmedizin* 51:839, 1975.

Chapter 10
Enhancing Health With Fiber

1. Burkitt D.P. And Trowell H.C. *Refined Carbohydrate Feeds the Disease: Some Implications of Dietary Fibre*. Academic Press: London and New York, 1975.

2. Painter N.S. *Diverticular Disease of the Colon*. Keats Publishing: New Canaan CT, 1975.

3. Anderson J. Talk given to the American Society of Contemporary Medicine and Surgery, 1991.

Chapter 12
The Longevity Potential of Yogurt

1. Walker M. *Secrets of Long Life*. Stamford CT: Freelance Publications, 1983.

2. Zurbel R. and Zurbel V. *The Vegetarian Family.* Englewood Cliffs NJ: Prentice-Hall, Inc., 1978, p. 123.

3 Sellars R.L. Health properties of yogurt. In R.C. Chandan (ed.): *Yogurt: Nutritional and Health Properties.* McLean VA: National Yogurt Association, 1989, pp. 115–144.

4. Chandan R.C. and Shahani K.M. Yogurt. In Y.H. Hui (ed.): *Dairy Science and Technology Handbook.* Vol. 2: Product Manufacturing. McLean VA: National Yogurt Association, 1993, pp. 10–11.

5. Metchnikoff E. *The Prolongation of Life.* New York: G.P. Putnam and Sons, The Knickerbocker Press, 1908.

6. Fernandes C.F. and Shahani K.M. Modulation of antibiosis by lactobacilli and yogurt and its healthful and beneficial significance. In R.C. Chandan (ed.): *Yogurt: Nutritional and Health Properties.* McLean VA: National Yogurt Association, 1989, pp. 145–159.

7. Gilliland S.E. and Speck M.L. Antagonistic action of *Lactobacillus acidophilus* toward intestinal and foodborne pathogens in associative cultures. *Journal of Food Prot* 40:820–823, 1977.

8. Hilton E. *Annals of Internal Medicine* 116:353, 1992.

9. *Acta Obstetricia et Gynecologica Scandinavica* 72:17, 1993.

10 DeSimone C.B., Salvadori B., Jirillo E., Baldinelli L., Bitonti F., and Vesely R. Modulation of immune activities in humans and animals by dietary lactic acid bacteria. In R.C. Chandan (ed.): *Yogurt: Nutritional and Health Properties.* McLean VA: National Yogurt Association, 1989, pp. 201–213.

11. Halpern G.M., Vruwink K.G., Van de Water J., Keen C.L., and Gershwin M.E. Influence of long-term yogurt consumption in young adults. *International Journal of Immunotherapy* 7(4):205–210, 1991.

12. *Foods, Nutrition and Immunity* 1:77, 1992.

13. *American Journal of Clinical Nutrition* 39:756, 1984.

14. *Journal of Dairy Science* 73:905, 1990.

Chapter 13
Using Chelation Therapy to Promote Longevity and Treat Alzheimer's Disease

1. Walker M. *The Chelation Way*. Garden City Park NY: Avery Publishing Group, 1990.

2. Walker M. *The Chelation Way*. Garden City Park NY: Avery Publishing Group, 1990.

3. Perl D.P. and Good P.F. The association of aluminum, Alzheimer's disease, and neurofibrillary tangles. *Journal of Neural Transm* [Suppl] 24:205–211, 1987.

4. Crapper-McLaughlan D.R.. McLachlan C.D., Krishnan B., Krishnan S.S., Dalton A.J., and Steele J.C. Aluminum and calcium in soil and food from Guam, Palau and Jamaica: implications for amyotrophic lateral sclerosis and parkinsonism-dementia syndromes of Guam. *Brain* 112:45–53, 1989.

5. Cranton E.M. *Bypassing Bypass*. Briarcliff Manor NY: Stein and Day, 1984, p. 84.

6. Crapper-McLachlan, D.R., Krishnan, S.S., and Quittkat, S. Aluminum, neurofibrillary degeneration, and Alzheimer's disease. *Brain* 99:68–80, 1976.

7. Balch J.F. and Balch P.A. *Prescription for Nutritional Healing*. 2nd ed. Garden City Park NY: Avery Publishing Group, 1997, p. 122.

8. Casdorph H.R. EDTA Chelation Therapy II: Efficacy in Brain Disorders. *Journal of Holistic Medicine* 3(2):101–117, Fall/Winter 1981.

Chapter 14
Restoring Vigor With Herbal Remedies

1. Shibata S., Tanaka O., Shoji J., and Saito H. Chemistry and pharmacology of panax. *Economic and Medicinal Plant Research* 1:217–284, 1985.

2. Balch J.F. and Balch P.A. *Prescription for Nutritional Healing*. 2nd ed. Garden City Park NY: Avery Publishing Group, 1997, pp. 54–55.

3. Fulder S. *The Ginseng Book.* Garden City Park NY: Avery Publishing Group, 1996, p. 24.

Chapter 15
Using Intravenous Hydrogen Peroxide to Fight Disease

1. Jay B.E., Finney J.W., Balla G.A., and others. The supersaturation of biologic fluids with oxygen by the decomposition of hydrogen peroxide. *Texas Reports of Biology and Medicine* 22:106–109, 1964.

2. Urschel H.C. Jr. Cardiovascular effects of hydrogen peroxide: current status. *Diseases of the Chest* 51:180–192, 1967.

3. Finney J.W., Jay B.E., Race G.J., and others. Removal of cholesterol and other lipids from experimental animal and human atheromatous arteries by dilute hydrogen peroxide. *Angiology* 17:223–228, 1966.

4. Mariani F. Le iniexioni endovence de casigeno nell' uomo. *Riforma Medecine* 18:194, 1902.

5. Tunnicliffe F.W. and Stebbing G.F. The intravenous injection of oxygen gas as a therapeutic measure. *Lancet* 11: 321–323, 1916.

6. Oliver T.H., Cantab B.C., and Murphy D.V. Influenzal pneumonia: the intravenous injection of hydrogen peroxide. *Lancet* 1:432–433, 1920.

7. Douglass W.C. *Hydrogen Peroxide, Medical Miracle.* Atlanta: Second Opinion Publishing, 1992.

8. Information from Drs. Elsasser, Morgan, and Stoesser was obtained at the First International Conference on Bio-Oxidative Medicine, September 1987.

Chapter 16
Fighting the Effects of Age With DHEA

1. Migeon C., Keller A., and Lawrence. DHEA and androsterone levels in human placenta. Effect of age and sex: day-

to-day and diurnal variations. *Journal of Clinical Endocrinology and Metabolism* 17:1051–1062, 1957.

2. Orentreich N., Brind J., Rizer R., and Vogelman J. Age changes and sex differences in serum dehydroepiandrosterone sulfate concentrations throughout adulthood. *Journal of Clinical Endocrinology and Metabolism* 59(3):551–554, 1984.

3. Wolkowitz O.M., Reus V.I., Roberts E., Manfredi F., Chan T., Ormiston S., Johnson R., Canick J., Brizendine L., and Weingartner J. Antidepressant and cognition-enhancing effects of DHEA in major depression. *Annals of the New York Academy of Science* 774:337–339, 1995.

4. Klatz R. and Goldman R. *DHEA: Stopping the Clock*. New Canaan CT: Keats Publishing, 1996.

5. Jesse R., Loesser K., Eich D., Qian Y.Z., Hess M.L., and Nestler J.E. Dehydroepiandrosterone inhibits human platelet aggregation *in vitro* and *in vivo*. *Annals of the New York Academy of Science* 774:281–290, 1995.

6. Haffa A.L., MacEwen E.G., Kurzman I.D., and Kemnitz J.W. Hypocholesterolemic effect of exogenous DHEA administration in the rhesus monkey. *In Vivo* 8(6):993–997, 1994.

7. Rich D.M., Nestler J.E., Johnson D.E., Dworkin G.H., Ko D., Wechsler A.S., and Hess M.L. Inhibition of accelerated coronary atherosclerosis with dehydroepiandrosterone in the heterotopic rabbit model of cardiac transplantation. *Circulation* 87(1):261–269, 1993.

8. Barrett-Conner E., Khaw K., and Yen S.C. A prospective study of dehydroepiandrosterone sulfate, mortality, and cardiovascular disease. *New England Journal of Medicine* 315:1519–1524, 1986.

9. Rasmussen K., Martin E., and Healey M. Effects of DHEA in immuno-suppressed rats infected with *Cryptosporidium parvum*. *Journal of Parasitology* 79(3):364–370, 1993.

10. Yen S.S., Morales A.J., and Khorram O. Replacement of DHEA in aging men and women. *Annals of the New York Academy of Science* 774:128–142, 1995.

11. Araneo B., Dowell T., Woods B., Daynes R., Judd M., and Evans T. DHEAS as an effective vaccine adjuvant in elderly humans. *Annals of the New York Academy of Science* 774:232–248, 1995.

12. Whitaker J. Be good to your mother (hormone, that is). *Health & Healing* 4(1), 1994.

13. Whitaker J. Be good to your mother (hormone, that is). *Health & Healing* 4(1), 1994.

14. Mulder J. and others. Dehydroepiandrosterone as predictor for progression to AIDS in asymptomatic human immunodeficiency virus type II infected men. *Journal of Immunodeficiency* 165:413–418, 1992.

15. Van Vollenhoven R. An open study of dehydroepiandrosterone in systemic lupus erythematosus. *Arthritis and Rheumatism* 37(9):1305–1310, 1994.

16. Nordin B. and others. The relationship between calcium absorption, serum DHEA, and vertebral mineral density in postmeopausal women. *Journal of Clinical Endocrinology and Metabolism* 60:651–657, 1985.

17. Taelman P. and others. Persistence of increased bone resorption and possible role of DHEA as a bone metabolism determinant in osteoporotic women in late postmenopause. *Maturitas* 11:65–73, 1989.

18. Casson P., Faquin L., Stentz F., Straughn A., Andersen R., Abraham G., and Buster J. Replacement of DHEA enhances T-lymphocyte insulin binding in postmenopausal women. *Fertility and Sterility* 63(5):1027–1031, 1995.

19. Bates C.W., Egerman R.S., Umstot E.S., Buster J.E., and Casson P.R. DHEA attenuates study-induced declines in insulin sensitivity in postmenopausal women. *Annals of the New York Academy of Science* 291–293, 1995.

20. Whitaker J. Obesity and diabetes. *Health & Healing* 2(11), 1992.

21. Cleary M.P. and others. Effect of DHEA on growth in

lean and obese Zucker rats. *Journal of Nutrition* 114:1242–1251, 1984.

22. Sahelian R. *DHEA: A Practical Guide.* Garden City Park NY: Avery Publishing Group, 1996, pp. 29–30.

23. Lucas J., Ahmed S.A., Casey L.M., and MacDonald P.C. Prevention of autoantibody formation and prolonged survival in New Zealand Black/New Zealand White F1 mice fed DHEA. *Journal of Clinical Investigation* 75:2091–2093, 1985.

24. Nestler J. DHEA: coming of age. *Annals of the New York Academy of Sciences* 774:ix–xi, 1995.

25. Morales A., Nolan J., Nelson J., and Yen S. Effects of replacement dose of DHEA in men and women of advancing age. *Journal of Clinical Endocrinology and Metabolism* 78: 1360–1367, 1994.

Chapter 17
The Gerovital Secret of Long Life

1. Walker M. *Secrets of Long Life.* Stamford CT: Freelance Communications, 1983.

2. Walker M. Secrets of *Los Viejos*—The Old Ones. *Townsend Letter for Doctors,* December 1992, pp. 1074–1077.

3. Airola P. *Rejuvenation Secrets From Around the World.* 1974, p. 51.

4. Sowemimo-Coker S.O., Yardin G., and Meiselman H.J. Effect of procaine hydrochloride on the aggregation behavior and suspension viscoelasticity of human red blood cells. *Biorheology* 26:951–972, 1989.

5. Zung W.W.K. and Wang H-S. Clinical trials of Gerovital H_3 in the treatment of depression in the elderly. *Geriatric Psychopharmacology* 346:233–246, 1979.

6. Aslan A. Procaine therapy in old age and other disorders (novocaine factor H_3). *Gerontology Clinics* 3:143, 1960.

7. Aslan A. The therapeutics of old age: the action of pro-

caine. In Bluemental H.T. (ed): *Medical and Clinical Aspects of Aging*. New York: Columbia University Press, 1962.

8. Aslan A., Vrabiescu A., Domilescu C., and others. Long-term treatment with procaine (Gerovital-H₃) in albino rats. *Journal of Gerontology* 20:1, 1965.

9. Verzar F. Note on the influence of procaine, PABA, and DEAE on the aging of rats. *Gerontologia* 3:351, 1959.

10. Smigel J.O., Piller J., Murphy C., and others. H₃ (procaine hydrochloride) therapy in aging institutionalized patients: an interim report. *Journal of the American Gerontological Society* 8: 785, 1960.

11. MacFarlane M.D. Procaine HCI (Gerovital-H₃): a weak, reversible, fully competitive inhibitor of monoamine oxidase. *Federation Proceedings* 34:1, 1975.

12. Zwerling I. Effects of a procaine preparation (Gerovital-H₃) in hospitalized geriatric patients: a double-blind study. *Journal of the American Geriatrics Society* 23:8, 1975.

13. Yau T.M. Gerovital-H₃, monoamine oxidases, and brain monoamine oxidase. In M. Rockstein (ed.): *Theoretical Aspects of Aging*. New York: Academic Press, 1974.

14. Hegner D. Pharmokinetic and pharmaco-dynamic aspects concerning procaine with special consideration of stabilization by hemaporphyrin. Symposium on procaine with stabilizer and preservative, Las Vegas, 10 July 1980.

15. Prokop L. A study of the capacity of orally administered procaine to improve performance. *Wiener Medizinische Wochenschrift* 123:658, 1973.

16. Doerling E. Maintenance of the efficiency level in older working people. *Der Kassenarzt* 19:2551–2555, 1975.

17. Hendler S.S. *The Complete Guide to Anti-Aging Nutrients*. New York: Simon and Schuster, 1985, pp. 285–287.

Index

A

Adaptation energy, 24
Addiction, 32–33
Aged garlic extract, 130
Aging
  and brain chemicals,
    32–33
  definitions of, 10
  effect of DHEA on,
    154–156
  effect of Gerovital on,
    159–163
  free radical theory of,
    11–12
  problem of, 10–11
  program to counteract,
    165–172
  role of antioxidants in,
    16–17
  role of brain allergies in,
    39

  role of mineral imbalance
    in, 49
  role of mineral toxicity
    in, 49
  role of stress reduction
    in, 29
Alfalfa, 56
Allergies, 32, 33
  anaphylactic, 37
  brain, 34–35, 37–39
  conventional treatment
    for, vs. clinical ecology,
    35–37, 38
Aloe, 110, 111
Aluminum toxicity, 126–127
Alzheimer's disease, chela-
    tion therapy and,
    126–127
American Academy of En-
    vironmental Medicine,
    36
Anderson, Dr. James, 97

K

Karaya, 108
Kelp, 56
Kidd, Dr. Parris, 64–65

L

Lactobacillus acidophilus, 118,
   119, 120
Lactobacillus bulgaricus, 117,
   120
Laxatives
   bulk-forming, 108–109
   lubricant, 112
   stimulant, 109–111
   stool-softener, 111–112
LDL. *See* Low density
   lipoprotein.
Life expectancy
   extending, 157–159
   in United States, 10
Lignins, 94
   food sources of, 99
   See also Fiber.
Lipofuscin, 13, 16
Locus ceruleus, 33
Lovage, 138
Low density lipoproteins,
   82, 97. *See also* Cholesterol.
Lung diseases, using
   hydrogen peroxide to
   treat, 146–147

M

Magnesium, 13, 48, 60–62,
   130. *See also* Antioxidants.
Malt soup extract, 108–109
Manganese, 130
   recommended daily
   amount of, 169
Masquelier, Dr. Jack, 89–90
Matsuura, Dr. Ustis, 42
McLachlan, Dr. Donald R.,
   127
Medicine, Chinese, 134–135
   herbal remedies, 135–139
   See also Medicine, herbal.
Medicine, herbal, rebirth of,
   133–135
Metchnikoff, Dr. Elias, 117
Methylcellulose, 108
Milk products, fermented,
   116. *See also* Yogurt.
Minerals
   functions of, 55–56
   in hair, significance of,
      44
   imbalance in, 47–49
   importance of, 54–56
   major, 53–62
   recommended daily
      amounts of, 169
   sources of, 56–57
   trace, 63–71
Monosodium glutamate
   (MSG), 36
Morgan, Dr. Kirk, 149

MSG. *See* Monosodium
glutamate.
Mucilage, 94
food sources of, 99
See also Fiber.
Myrrh, 136

N

N, N-dimethyl-glycine. *See*
DMG.
National Institute of Geron-
tologic Research and
Geriatric Medicine,
159
Niacin, 81–86
function of, 81–83
supplements, and chromi-
um, 83–86
Niacinamide, 83, 83
Norepinephrine, 33
Nung, Shen, 134, 135

O

Oligomeric proantho-
cyamidins. *See* OPC.
OPC, 89–92

P

Painter, Dr. Neil, 96
Pantothenic acid, recom-
mended daily amount
of, 169

Pectin, 94
food sources of, 99
See also Fiber.
Pen Ching, 135
Pepper, black, 139
Peppermint, 141
Perl, Dr. Daniel, 126–127
Peroxides, 11, 15–16
Phosphorus, 59–60
Pollution, 74
as cause of allergies, 38
Polycarbophil, 109
Potassium, recommended
daily amount of, 169
Pregnenolone, 155
Prickly ash, 141–142
Privet, 138
Prolongation of Life, The, 117
Protomorphogens, 131
Prune concentrate dehy-
drate, 110
Psyllium preparations, 109
Pyridoxine, 82
recommended daily
amount of, 169

R

Radio-allergo-sorbent test,
36, 37
RAST. *See* Radio-allergo-sor-
bent test.
RDA. *See* Recommended
Dietary Allowance.
Recommended Dietary Al-
lowance, 53

Vitamin B12. *See* Cobalamin.

Vitamin C, 13, 16, 48
and antioxidants, 87–89
as oral chelator, 129
using, with antioxidants, 92
See also Antioxidants.

Vitamin D3, recommended daily amount of, 169

Vitamin E, 13, 15–16, 48
deficiency of, 12–13
as oral chelator, 129
recommended daily amount of, 169
See also Antioxidants.

VLDL. *See* Very low density lipoprotein.

W

Wax, 94. *See also* Fiber.
White poplar, 136
Wolfberry, 139

Y

Yogurt, 116–122

Z

Zinc, 48, 67–69, 130